A Journey of One

Hospice: Healing and Teaching by Storytelling

A.L. CROMWELL, RN

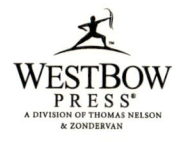

WESTBOW
PRESS®
A DIVISION OF THOMAS NELSON
& ZONDERVAN

Copyright © 2019 A.L. Cromwell, RN.

All rights reserved. No part of this book may be used or reproduced by any means, graphic, electronic, or mechanical, including photocopying, recording, taping or by any information storage retrieval system without the written permission of the author except in the case of brief quotations embodied in critical articles and reviews.

This book is a work of non-fiction. Unless otherwise noted, the author and the publisher make no explicit guarantees as to the accuracy of the information contained in this book and in some cases, names of people and places have been altered to protect their privacy.

WestBow Press books may be ordered through booksellers or by contacting:

WestBow Press
A Division of Thomas Nelson & Zondervan
1663 Liberty Drive
Bloomington, IN 47403
www.westbowpress.com
1 (866) 928-1240

Because of the dynamic nature of the Internet, any web addresses or links contained in this book may have changed since publication and may no longer be valid. The views expressed in this work are solely those of the author and do not necessarily reflect the views of the publisher, and the publisher hereby disclaims any responsibility for them.

Any people depicted in stock imagery provided by Getty Images are models, and such images are being used for illustrative purposes only. Certain stock imagery © Getty Images.

THE HOLY BIBLE, NEW INTERNATIONAL VERSION®, NIV® Copyright © 1973, 1978, 1984, 2011 by Biblica, Inc.® Used by permission. All rights reserved worldwide.

ISBN: 978-1-9736-7822-9 (sc)
ISBN: 978-1-9736-7823-6 (hc)
ISBN: 978-1-9736-7821-2 (e)

Library of Congress Control Number: 2019917260

Print information available on the last page.

WestBow Press rev. date: 12/10/2019

Lovingly dedicated to the concept of hospice
and the care of the terminally ill in a family care setting,

and to those in the grind who make it happen.

Also dedicated to my father, Dr. C. Phil Cheatham,
who, in his never-ending thirst for understanding of
God and life, lovingly and without fear shared with
me his thoughts and dying experiences as they were
occurring. I love you, Dad. I'm passing it on.

CONTENTS

Note to the Reader: How to Read This Book ix
Acknowledgments xi
A Journey of One: *For the Caregiver* xiii
What Is Hospice? xv
Note from the Author xvii

Chapter 1: Henry's Journey 1
    Questions for Reflection 20
Chapter 2: Tracy's Journey 21
    Questions for Reflection 39
Chapter 3: Jon's Journey 40
    Questions for Reflection 59
Chapter 4: Martina's Journey 60
    Questions for Reflection 86
Chapter 5: Zoe's Journey 87
    Questions for Reflection 109
Chapter 6: The "Loved One" 110
    Dream Vision: What It's Like for Me 110
    Questions for Reflection 117

References 119
    Family Calendar 119
    Palliative Performance Scale (PPS) 120
    Karnofsky Performance Status (KPS) 121
    FAST Scale: Functional Assessment Staging Tool
    for Dementia 122
    Sharing the Gospel Story with Your Loved One 123
    Life Review with Your Loved One 125

NOTE TO THE READER
HOW TO READ THIS BOOK

This book is written to give practical advice to those caring for an ill loved one, with the additional purpose of beginning the healing process for those of us left behind. But sometimes the pain is too fresh or the time is just not right. Most will find this a book to be visited and revisited, rather than to be read through in a single sitting. If sadness overflows, set the book down and visit with your memories. There is much greater healing in this action than in the reading of a book.

Suggestions for Reading

- Skim the *text box topics* to find the information that you need right now.

- Answer the *Questions for Reflection* to break the ice.

- Read only the chapter that pertains to your loved one's diagnosis.

- Skip to chapters 5 and 6 if you are feeling emotionally overwhelmed.

- If it hurts more than helps, set it down! Pick it up again later after some healing time has passed.

ACKNOWLEDGMENTS

A beloved thank-you to my husband, Kyle, who shows me daily how to love and honor God, keeps us focused on the bigger picture, and makes my life spark.

To my children, Elizabeth and Steven, you complete my life, and you are my joy.

To my brother and sister, Chuck and Lauren, who always support me in every endeavor; you have taught me everything about how a family can pull together in the hard times.

To my deceased mother and brothers, Adrienne, Phil Jr. and Ben, your struggles and victories are woven within these pages.

To the following specialists who helped me hone and explain the concepts of hospice:

> Eric D. Blakney, MD, HMPC, Board Certified in Internal Medicine, Certified in Hospice and Palliative Care Medicine, Hospice Medical Director Certified
>
> R. James Burnett, DO, Board Certified in Family Medicine, Certified in Addictive Diseases by the American Society of Addiction Medicine (ASAM), Retired
>
> Frank Calder, PharmD, Retired
>
> Sam Shaw, Jr., DMin, MDiv, Pastor
>
> Michelle Tipton, RN, Hospice Director of Operations
>
> Gosta Turman, RN, Hospice Clinical Manager
>
> Nancy Hoover, CPNP, APRN, RN, CLC
>
> Mary Beth Miller, RN

Terri Steward, MSN, RN

AnnieLaurie Walters, Communications Consultant

To the Memphis hospice team, you are not just my coworkers, you are my heroes.

A special thank-you to "Zoe" and her family, who came into my life at a critical time in the writing of this book. Their willingness to share their hearts, their pain, and their lives with me helped define the mission of this book.

A JOURNEY OF ONE

FOR THE CAREGIVER

Hospice is a word associated with darkened rooms and deathbeds, nun-like nurses, and sorrowful mourners at closed doors. It's a word that means "I am so sorry" and "I suppose it won't be long now." Death is disquieting, even for those of us who make our living accompanying it from door to door. *But death is frequently misinterpreted, as I hope you will discover through these stories.* It is not an end, but a destination, a journey down a singular road, right to the face of God. And the body knows how to get there. Since its birth, it has been preprogrammed for this. There is a process, a predictability. Yet the last breath of this earth, the cessation of life in a loved one, still comes as a surprise to us. Apparently, we can never truly "prepare" for it. Knowing how it has looked for others and what they have experienced along the way, however, may provide some comfort and reassurance for you and for your loved one, as you accompany him or her on the pilgrimage: the journey of one.

This book has been compiled from many hospice experiences and from many hospice providers and caregivers. It is not meant to give medical advice nor give direction as to how your hospice agency should perform its duties in the care of your loved one. *Its purpose is only to share a few stories with you, with the hope that you will not feel alone at this difficult time.* Caring for another on this road is one of the greatest honors that a loved one can bestow—the ultimate sacrifice of your time for theirs. These stories are written in honor of all caregivers who have essentially contracted with their loved ones to walk alongside them during their dying process. It is a relationship of new depth, one that is usually reserved for impersonal hospital rooms, fluorescent lighting, and uniformed strangers. Hospice in the home can be a difficult undertaking, sometimes for the dying and always for the caregiving. Your story will have long-term value, however. You will discover this value in your day-by-day walk, and it will come back to you again when you see others start the journey with their loved ones, simply because you walked it first.

It's a lost art, dying at home. Since the dissolution of the multifamily home, death has become an institutional process. But not too long ago, caring for a relative or neighbor who was passing from this world to the next was a family event. The conversations may have been hushed and sorrowful, but everyone was involved in the care, even small children, who learned to bring a cup of water or an extra blanket. These children, now the "baby boomers," are approaching their later years, and this has created a change in the concept of hospice. It is no longer for the last days or weeks of a person's life, and it doesn't have to mean, "Oh, I'm so sorry." Some recipients of hospice are still employed at their jobs. Others are placed on hospice and then improve, having been chronically ill rather than terminally ill. Some who start out at home are eventually placed in nursing homes or hospice facilities. There are many hospice stories that may surprise you, and many that will heal or inspire you. Come join us on our journey of care, helping others to walk their journey of one.

WHAT IS HOSPICE?

Hospice refers to the care of the terminally ill in a family-centered setting. It may occur in a home or in a facility, depending on family preference and resources. Hospice care is covered by most insurances and includes physician services, nursing services, equipment, supplies, and basic medications related to comfort. It also offers aide, chaplain, and social work support. Some hospice agencies provide volunteer services, and all have access to dietary counseling and short-term physical and occupational therapy. Short-term inpatient and respite care are also available, as well as long-term bereavement services for the caregivers and family. The purpose of hospice is to provide comfort and dignity for the patient and to promote quality of life through the very end of life. Family, quality of life, and terminal illness do not seem like mutual companions, but as many have discovered, they truly can be intertwined. Where quantity and longevity diminish, quality flourishes.

You are about to enter a world of new concepts. Each day will bring a new and sometimes difficult conversation. There will be more losses than gains. There are moments of awkwardness and times when obstacles cannot be overcome. There is an inherent element of trauma bonding. There are no clear paths or maps available, only a vague trail marked with suggestions and encouragements from others: "This has worked for some" or "Let's try this other for a while." Sometimes you will be at an absolute loss and can only sit down next to your loved one and wait for something different to happen. You will learn that most issues cannot be fixed and that many expectations will not be met. There may be few days when you don't fall into bed exhausted, frustrated, and feeling helpless. This will be a full-time but temporary job. Just as birthing a baby into this world is not an easy task, assisting with the passing of a human into the next world is the same. Both come with pain and reward. May this book bring you the courage to venture on this path and embrace this journey together—you, your loved one, your family, and your hospice team.

NOTE FROM THE AUTHOR

I expect that this will be a small-audience book. But for those who read its pages and have committed to sharing in the care of their loved one's final days, you are my heroes. For some, it will be a natural undertaking. You've seen it before, or perhaps you have been blessed with the inherent gift of caregiving. For others, the struggle will be a difficult one. Do I wish for you that this will be an abbreviated struggle? In a way, yes. Losing a loved one is often the hardest event of an entire lifetime, and there are never enough days with them—never. But if this life is the vapor and the next life is the true life, might we amend our desire to hold them on the path and instead bless them on it? The timing, anyway, is apparently not ours to appoint.

Why tell hospice stories?

When my children were young, I weighed the option of homeschooling them during their critical foundational years. I purchased a curriculum and scoured the proposed schedule and teaching points, but I could not extract from these what a real day would look like. The responsibility seemed daunting. Did I have what it would take to fill the shoes? It was my sister-in-law who affirmed for me that I could indeed homeschool. She tutored me not by lecture or review but by simply telling me the stories of her own homeschooling experiences. We shared many glasses of iced tea that summer, talking while our children played, and by the end of it, I was ready to teach. I *felt* like a homeschool teacher, simply from hearing her stories. I didn't do it perfectly—just ask my children. But together we accomplished it, usually muddling, often plodding, sometimes inspired. And we were wonderfully blessed by the journey together. After a few years, my children returned to traditional school, and I returned to my nursing job. Our homeschool path had been a full-time but temporary endeavor.

This collection of hospice stories is designed to teach by storytelling. Or if your loved one has already passed, perhaps it will give you some closure, knowing that what you saw and experienced was a part of a larger, fully natural event.

Your hospice experiences will all be different. But this fact will not change: it *will* be a full-time and temporary undertaking. Eventually, your paths will disentangle, and you will resume your individual ways—you will return to your life, and your loved one will go on to his or hers.

May God bless you both on your journeys,
Leigh

Why, you do not even know what will happen tomorrow. What is your life? You are a mist that appears for a little while and then vanishes.
—James 4:14

My Father's house has many rooms; if that were not so, would I have told you that I am going there to prepare a place for you? And if I go and prepare a place for you, I will come back and take you to be with me that you also may be where I am. You know the way to the place where I am going.
—John 14:2–4

CHAPTER 1

Henry's Journey

- Age 76, heart failure
- Primary symptoms: weakness and fatigue
- Primary caregivers: Lynette (32) and Daniel (43)

The Road Together

Henry and His Family

Henry L. Sherman is a seventy-six-year-old male with end-stage heart failure. He is a retired architect by trade and lives in the original home that he designed for his wife of fifty-five years. Together, they raised four children who are now grown but still live nearby—something their mother had been insistent upon. Family had been important to her, and Henry is grateful for the full life they created together. Henry enjoys the daily visits from one or another child, his grandchildren, and even his great-grandchildren, although the visits are often brief, as everyone is busy. Lynette, his youngest, stops by most often. But only Daniel, the still-single one, is able to fully adjust his schedule for Henry's lengthier needs. Daniel shops for groceries, buys clothes, and picks up meals from the family's favorite restaurant. In fact, Daniel will do anything for his dad—except doctor's appointments. He has always been the first to gag at a dirty diaper or vomit at the sight of blood. Obvious to the rest of the family, Daniel never raised children.

Mrs. Sherman has been gone two years now, and the children have begged their father to move in with one of them. But Henry loves the old home and treasures the memories that surround him. His whole life is here, in every wall decoration and whatnot. Every picture on the mantle and on every flat surface of the house represents a day of happiness and fulfillment to him. He is content to spend his present in the past and wonders only a little about what's ahead.

A Bad Heart

Henry has been aware of his heart condition for several years, but his wife's care had taken precedence. He was slowing down, he knew, and his balance was off. A few months ago, Henry had taken a bad fall. Fortunately, he had been close enough to reach the coiled cord of the old wall phone and had been able to call an ambulance. No bones were broken, but that was the only good news from the hospital visit that day. The results of Henry's tests showed a significant decline in cardiac function, which was the cause of the dizziness and balance issues. It also accounted for the swelling in his ankles and the extra pillows he required to sleep at night. The emergency room doctor adjusted Henry's medications, and he had been sent home with a walker and a warning that future falls could be expected.

The children had petitioned, but Henry once again refused to move, so a paid caregiver had been engaged to help—to the limited degree that Henry would consent. She used her own key in the mornings, helping Henry out of bed and assisting him with his morning care, and then thankfully leaving him to spend his afternoons sunk in his recliner and memories. She returned in the evenings to help him back to bed, where he slept heavily until morning.

As forecasted by the doctor, Henry's condition declined, and within six months Henry was living a basic bed-to-chair existence, spending his days and often entire nights in his recliner. He was still able to walk from room to room using the cumbersome walker, but he chose less and less often to make the trip. He preferred chips and cookies to the meals that his children prepared for him, as, he argued stubbornly, they were easy to fix and tasted good.

Home health was arranged, but Henry became short of breath with the simplest of exercises, and to his relief, the therapy was discontinued. His self-motivation in general was wavering. "But that's just what happens to old people," Henry told his children, having seen it himself in his own parents and grandparents. They remained insistent and cajoling, however, quarreling amongst themselves about what was best for their father. They did not know whether this was truly a bad heart stealing their dad's energy or whether he was just giving up. Henry was approaching a crossroads.

The Path Bends

Dad's Dying?

It was the caregiver who found Henry on the floor this time. He appeared to be only bumped and bruised again, but the hospital ran him through their tests anyway. His cardiac results returned with dangerously low scores, and his oxygen levels had dropped another tier. There was no doubt about it in the eyes of the doctors—Henry's heart was losing strength. The cardiologist was thorough in his explanation that Henry's weakness and fatigue were not choices but was instead a status change brought on by a failing heart.

| A slow decline |

And then the cardiologist spoke the word: *hospice.*

"You mean he's dying?" Lynette was shocked by the word. She knew her father was in his later years, but surely, he had several more to go. He just wasn't trying hard enough. Maybe if he exercised more? The doctor, careful of his words, explained the test results again and recapped the symptoms that Henry had experienced over the past year. He explained that hospice did not necessarily mean that her father was dying right away; hospice also included the months of care prior to death. Lynette felt little reassured by this.

"So how much time does he have?" she asked, shaken, looking over at her father. Henry, worn out from the day's events, was sleeping heavily. The doctor pulled his chair closer to hers for the explanation.

Qualifications for Hospice Care

"There are general courses that most diseases follow," he began, "although the outcomes do vary. It is my belief that your father is terminally ill and that the expected course of his disease will most likely cause his death within six months."

Certificate of Terminal Illness

He went on to explain that while Mr. Sherman would not get any better, there was certainly the possibility that he might live longer than six months. They could only look at general symptoms of his disease and project an outcome by the pattern of decline that Mr. Sherman had been displaying up to this point. Since he appeared to be on a slow decline rather than a fast fall, the doctor was hopeful that this slow pattern would continue.

"Hospice can help him enjoy a substantial quality of life in whatever time he has left, Lynette. Since there is nothing else that can be done for his improvement, this is our goal, however many weeks or months he may have."

Starting hospice care early

Lynette caught the words—weeks or months and not years.

The doctor went on, "He will remain under a doctor's care, and the hospice staff is specially trained in end-of-life conditions. They will be in his home much more often than if he were coming to my office. We have done everything we can for him, Lynette. There are no more medications or treatments to try. I'm afraid that his heart is just running down. If I'm wrong and it turns out that his condition is indeed chronic rather than terminal, hospice will discharge him and we'll return to what we're doing now. I doubt that this is the case, but we can always hope for that. In any matter, I like to get my patients into hospice early, in case things take a turn for the worse. It's always better to be prepared rather than surprised. I have a hospice agency that I tend to refer patients to, but you can choose your own, of course. If you're on board with this, I'm going to review his medications and discontinue any that aren't absolutely necessary. We need to keep all functions available for the main fight now. I'll send in my nurse to answer any other questions you may have."

Lynette nodded absently, still dazed by the seemingly sudden turn of events. The doctor left, and the room was quiet. Her father snored, his wrinkles relaxed. His face was a pale gray in the hospital lighting. She sat, hands gripped tightly in her lap, trying to understand what she had just heard. *Hospice. Six months. No more hospitals. Nothing left to try.*

Hospice Referral

Eventually, a nurse arrived with discharge papers, the order for hospice care fluttering at the top of the stack. She spoke briskly. "The doctor believes that Mr. Sherman is no longer safe to stay at home by himself, so we'll need to know where he's going in order to coordinate his equipment and hospice services."

Lynette glanced nervously over at her father and wondered, *Did he hear that? No, gratefully he was still asleep.*

The nurse noted the concern and amended her course. Apparently, this news was not expected.

"I'm so sorry," she said. "This must be new information for you. Let me see if I can answer your questions. My mother was on hospice a few years ago. Maybe I can help you with some decisions. What concerns are you having?" She slowed her pace, handing over the folders to Lynette, and then sat down in the extra chair.

She clasped her hands loosely, waiting for Lynette to collect her thoughts. Lynette's many apprehensions were evident in the way she stared at the ominous referral paper clipped to the discharge folder.

"How much is hospice going to cost?" she asked, somewhat embarrassed. "Dad doesn't have much money left after Mother's cancer. And the rest of us are raising our families. Will it be expensive?"

"Hospice services will be covered by his insurance, so there is no cost to him," the nurse explained, "as long as you don't pursue any diagnostic or curative treatments, which the doctors have agreed aren't helpful anymore. The hospice agency can answer coverage questions more specifically. I remember how hard it can be to make this mental jump, to move from 'Let's fix it' to 'Let them enjoy their last days.'"

The nurse's gaze lowered to the floor for a moment, returning to the day she was told that her mother's road was turning.

"How often will hospice be there?" Lynette asked next, bringing the nurse back to the present issue. "Will they stay with him all day?" She was inwardly cringing at how busy they all were with their own families. The nurse shared the basics with her.

"The role of hospice is to manage your father's comfort and care needs, but they don't provide the role of caregiver. Just like with our children, general insurances don't pay for sitters and caregiver services. The hospice team will manage his case and see to his medical needs. They will give him a brief physical exam each visit, check his medications and supplies, and address any new needs that have arisen. Their aides will give him a bath, usually a few times a week. A social worker and chaplain will also visit, and some agencies also have volunteer services. Some have hospices houses as well, which are residential facilities that do provide the daily care needs, similar to what a nursing home provides. If the patient remains at home, then the daily care and supervision must be furnished by the family. Family care is what usually occurs in times of illness, though we're not often prepared for it. Our

Hospice and the family caregiver

social worker can help you with nursing home placement if you'd rather. The room and board would need to be paid for in the usual manner …" but Lynette was shaking her head.

"We don't want him in a nursing home. I'm sure we'll figure it out somehow." She thought of the family home, hoping they would not have to sell it. Their mother's illness had depleted the retirement savings, and her father's Social Security was barely covering his monthly bills. She gazed out the window, clutching the hospital packet in her hands. But the hospice referral was all that her mind could see.

Discharge Decisions

The nurse realized that Mr. Sherman's daughter was having trouble listening, much less making decisions, so she suggested a first step.

"Let's keep things simple," she offered. "Just start with what you know now. Call your family and decide where your father will stay for the next few days; you can always make changes later. Hospice isn't tied to a location, so they can provide his care anywhere, even in a nursing facility if you do decide on that route. They can help, Lynette, and they come to him, wherever he is. In the meantime, I'll arrange for our social worker to come speak with you. Then I'll come back and help you make discharge arrangements." She left the room, resting a hand for a moment on Lynette's shoulder before walking out, but Lynette was not aware. She was wondering how to tell the family.

Hospice is not limited by location.

Making It Work

Lynette's siblings were mixed in their reactions, but they cooperated enough to get through the next few days. Dad would go back to his home with twenty-four-hour paid caregiver services through the weekend, while the family met to decide what to do next. The hospital social worker had advised that six people were generally needed to care for a terminally ill person in the home, to guard against caregiver burnout. The family counted heads and concluded that they could maintain half of the care hours themselves and would have to pool resources for the rest. When they tallied the financial costs, however, it became clear that further compromise was needed. They decided to reach out to the hospice agency, not to sign yet, but to get added advice.

A hospice nurse arrived that evening. After a physical assessment and conversation with Mr. Sherman, the nurse convened with the family members in the den. She described the hospice program much as the doctor and hospital nurse had but added some additional tips. There may be medications that hospice would now cover that Mr. Sherman had been paying for himself, especially those related to his comfort. The family would no longer require days off work for doctor's appointments, though the family calculated that the increase of his care hours might counterbalance that particular savings. Hospice would supply many of Mr. Sherman's personal care items, and a hospice aide could be sent out for his bath so perhaps their private sitter might consider adjusting her fee. Most home equipment, such as hospital beds and oxygen, would be covered, so personal rental would not be necessary. The nurse concluded with a message similar to the one given by the hospital staff: in times of illness, all lives change, at least for a while.

The family conferred again and could only agree that they didn't want to use a nursing home if it could be avoided. Everything else remained in confusion and uncertainty. But there was no cost to this program, and the information was consistent, so the papers were signed. Mr. Sherman was now on hospice.

Everybody Pitches In

Family discussions continued, and confusion slowly cleared as the hospice staff came to make their assessments over the next several days. With the encouragement and education of each staff member, the siblings became increasingly more comfortable with the prospect of caring for their father in his home. Much of their reticence had originated from fear rather than actual inability. With the help of the hospice social worker, they worked out a family calendar, splitting the days into shifts that worked around their crazy job schedules, school schedules, and kids' activity schedules. Daniel offered to provide the lion's share of the hours, but all were concerned about his weak stomach when it came to "gross things." For now, however, they were grateful for his availability. Friends and church members were called in as well, and the family pooled their money to pay for shifts that were not voluntarily covered.

> Caregiving: a full-time, temporary job

It was encouraging to see Henry actually improve over the next several weeks due to the sudden influx of company and the tweaking of care management by the hospice staff. His appetite improved, and he enjoyed hot meals with his family at the dinner table again. His house was cleaned during his children's shifts, and his papers and bills were organized. And for the most part, Henry was happy for the company and the help.

Better, but Not Perfect

Even though Henry's living and social conditions improved, all was not rosy. Henry often disagreed with his children's supervision, reminding them that he was a full-grown adult and twice their age. He complained that he should be able to sleep and wake when he wanted to, and he grumbled that they fretted over him too much. And Mr. Henry L. Sherman expressed himself fully and grandly on the day the children sold his car. They pointed out that they needed the money to provide for his care, but all Henry could see was the control of his life persistently and steadily being removed.

The First Diaper Change

More difficult conversations came when Henry could no longer get up to the bedside commode, even with help. The agency sent out adult diapers, but Henry would have none of it. He had diapered his children's backsides, but they would not diaper his. Oddly, it was Daniel who found the way, using a little respectful humor. He came whistling into his father's bedroom one morning, baby wipes in one hand and a wash basin in the other, an adult diaper fastened on top of his jeans and a clothespin on his nose. He told his father cheerfully that today was "payback time." Henry argued, as expected, but eventually Daniel knelt down by the bed and spoke earnestly into his father's knotted face, his own countenance wavering.

> *A labor of love*

"Dad, you know that I'm the last one to be able to do this, but no one else has the guts to face you on this. It's either us or the nursing home, and we like having you here. Can you try to bear it and allow me to do this for you? We'll sing a manly song, we'll both gag, and then it'll be done." Henry, at a loss, finally grunted his consent, and the diaper job got done to the tune of "One Hundred Bottles of Beer on the Wall." The next time was easier, taking only sixty bottles.

🍃 The Crossroads 🍃

Despite the family's intensified care, Henry gradually slipped back to his previous state, sleeping more and eating less. The weight he'd gained in the past year of inactivity fell off in striking measure. The swelling in his legs worsened, his toes and ankles progressing from dusky white to dark blue. Diuretic doses were adjusted, but nothing could overcome the sluggishness of Henry's failing heart.

The diuretics made for more diaper changes, but the family, sharing the night shifts while still working their day jobs, allowed their father to sleep through the night. When redness appeared on the thinning skin of Henry's sacrum, the nurse called a family huddle. She was quick to decline their request for a catheter, explaining that these become easy roadways for bacteria to travel up to the bladder and that Mr. Sherman's weakened immune system could not handle the barrage of urinary tract infections that would surely follow. The only answer was to change his diaper more frequently, and she would order a heavier barrier cream for the diaper changes. Henry's oldest daughter designed a meal plan for her father that included nutrient-dense foods and proteins for his skin, but Henry's burgeoning loss of interest in food included with it any true intent of improving his health. He began asking for his favorite chips and cookies again, ignoring the urgings to eat what was "good for him."

This new dilemma brought further conferences with the nurse, who proposed a principle known as pleasure eating. She explained that no diet could overcome a failing physical system, so it was an acceptable practice to allow a person to choose what he wanted to eat during the last phase of his life, the intent being a focus on quality of life rather than simple longevity. They considered this proposal and eventually all agreed. The oldest still offered protein shakes, and Daniel still offered Oreos, but they no longer argued with their father or with each other about which was right or best.

> Eating for comfort

Skin Care and Bedsores

The family began setting their clocks at night, adding additional diaper changes at the persistence of the nurse, who was aware of how quickly bedsores could progress. Skin breakdown prevention became the new battle line. The nurse reinforced the hospice aide's

> More labor, more love

demonstration of positioning Mr. Sherman with pillows and bolsters. Together, they taught the family how to use a draw-sheet to turn Mr. Sherman every two hours, so that no areas remained pressed into the bed mattress too long, as it was this restriction of blood supply that created most bedsores. But despite their efforts, Henry developed shallow ulcers on his hips and buttocks. The agency increased their skilled nurse visits for wound care, and the family received instruction in the cleaning of wounds and the changing of dressings—more new territory for them. But by this time, they had solidified into a dedicated family team and were of a common purpose. Their father was getting closer to his end, and they realized that their labor of love would have an eventual end as well. In the meantime, however, all were approaching their limits. Jobs were suffering, families were faltering, and homes were functioning on bare basics.

Sacrificing Self

The grandchildren were recruited next, not all willingly. They were taught the cleaning of bathrooms and kitchens, the folding of laundry, and the preparation of simple meals. And at Granddad's house, they acquired more new skills. They learned to raise the head of his bed before giving him a sip of water. They spent long afternoons at his house so that parents could monitor their homework and their play. Henry was asleep much of the day by then, but when he woke to see a grandchild sitting by his bedside, his smile made all their hardships worth their effort. His family was beside him, and that made Henry happy. He decided to forgive them for the car thing.

And the grandchildren learned something else, a thing far more significant than just the giving of a sip of water. They were witnessing a more important value—to sometimes sacrifice your life for another's need. One grandchild had dropped out of soccer because there were no available parents to drive her to the practices. Others were forced to give up their social activities as well. Some of them found the loosened supervision to be freeing and took advantage; others found it to be an opportunity for growth, and they matured and deepened in character. This episode of their lives was certainly more challenging than the controlled chaos that had been their life prior to their grandfather's illness. In fact, it was adding third and fourth layers of disorder. But something more crucial and life-changing was being anchored, something that soccer practice and report cards could not provide.

A Journey of One

What Is Henry Experiencing?

As Henry's time drew nearer, his family sought out the hospice staff to ask what their father might be experiencing. What was it like for him? They noticed that when he was awake his mind seemed generally clear, though very little of his natural energy was present. And he seemed to be withdrawing more and more each day. He mumbled and talked often in his sleep, and there were suspicions that he might be seeing people who were not present. Was he just dreaming, or was he really seeing others? Was he afraid of dying, as they were afraid of losing him? And what would he experience as he died?

Friends and family tried to interpret these unanswerable questions, but the hospice chaplain provided the most reassurance. During his assessment visit, the chaplain asked Henry if he had a faith.

"Not a 'religion,' Henry," the chaplain clarified, "but a belief that there is a God who has a place for you to go after you pass from this world."

The response from Henry, and repeated often by his family, was that he was tired, and he just wanted to be with his wife. He seemed to have an understanding that she was waiting for him. He would explain, when he had the energy, that he didn't

> *What does my loved one feel?*

know what that part looked like exactly, just that he felt their mother was nearby. And he assured them many times over that he was not afraid, that he knew somehow that everything was going to be all right. Some still worried, of course, unsure if this was his mind going or perhaps it was the medications talking. But hopefully, prayerfully, the sense of peace he seemed to have was real.

A further interpretation came a few evenings later, as the on-call nurse sat with them, waiting to see if the new dose of anxiety medication would ease Henry's now prevalent shortness of breath. Over a cup of coffee, she shared her own understanding, bringing in her knowledge of the physical phenomena that accompanied death. She prefaced her conversation with this statement:

"As a nurse, I have a scientific perspective," she explained, "and I research everything before I make a conclusion. But I'm also a person of faith, so I'm aware of ways that the two unite. We do not have proof of what happens to us after we die, but we know a little better now what happens to some of us *as* we die."

Lynette and Daniel were the only ones present for this discourse, the hour being late and the others having left. But these were the main seekers of answers, both trying to find something deeper in this dark ordeal and wrestling for an unfound peace of their own.

The Physical Phenomenon of Dying

The nurse shared with them several stories of near-death experiences, explaining that these experiences were the closest that we could come to understanding what happens to us as we die. Daniel cut in with a dismissal that these crazy stories were too outlandish to be taken seriously, and the nurse nodded in agreement that we should always question and search further.

"But with two thousand experiences now compiled on the internet," she pressed, "there are some consistencies that appear to be plausible, simply because of their statistical value.

"My scientific side questions the bizarre nature of it as well," she went on. "But my faith side tells me that sometimes things are true."

She raised an eyebrow to Daniel, tagging him to see if he wished her to go on. Daniel tipped his head as a signal to continue, inwardly hoping that she wouldn't get too spiritual. He had to acknowledge, however, that he was hoping for news that could make him feel a little better about this death watch. He needed to bring some light into these lonely days of watching his father slowly die. So he waited as the nurse took a sip of her coffee and spoke on.

"In the majority of the accounts, the person who passes is fully conscious and remains alert during the dying event, not experiencing 'death' at all—more like a leaving, or a 'lifting out.' They generally describe an essence of goodness, of well-being. Things are crisper, clearer, fully understood. And when they find themselves returned abruptly to their body, the consistent response is one of intense regret at being forced back. Even those who had full and gratifying lives say they preferred to remain in that new nature, rather than being returned to their body."

She then explained the physical hormones and chemicals that are released when organ systems begin their shutdown.

"We call them toxins," she defined for them, "which sounds distressing, but they are actually natural chemicals that act as painkillers and hallucinogens. These are serotonins, endorphins, natural melatonin, and several others. One in particular, dimethyltryptamine, is getting a great deal of new attention because of its psychedelic effects on the brain. Whether you believe that God gives you peace directly, or that God designed the chemicals in your body that release and give you the peace, or that there is no God and the chemicals are just there, it all comes to the same conclusion—the body knows how to die, and it does it well. And apparently, we make the journey on a cloud nine!" Her lips turned up in a bit of a smile, but she governed it, not wanting

> Natural pain relievers

A Journey of One

to be disrespectful of the gravity of the current situation. The family members in front of her were experiencing the dying of a loved one, and discussing the physiology of death could draw a fine line. Sometimes, it comforted, but just as often, it distressed. She assessed the nonverbal cues that she saw in the two listeners and decided to continue, even though the next was by far the riskier story to share.

> *What you are seeing is not what they are experiencing*

"Can we go offline a bit?" she asked, gambling.

Lynette and Daniel both nodded, their curiosity piqued by the question.

"I'm going to apologize for the graphic nature of this next story, but it does give credence to the information I just shared with you." She asked their permission once again and then proceeded. She recalled to them a rare but peculiar activity that was often reported quietly in the news as a suicide attempt.

"These are incidents in which participants self-strangulate and then release the rope from their necks just before death overtakes them."

She explained to them that these were not suicide seekers but were usually experienced drug users, ones who were especially well-versed in their trade. They had experimented with multiple combinations of drugs and substances, and the repeated explanation for their risky and ill-advised behavior was that the natural high of near-death was so extraordinary and so unimaginable—so far above any other high—that it could not be achieved with man-made chemicals. What they would feel, as systems were closing down, was worth the risk of never returning from it.

Daniel and Lynette sat stunned by the difficult story, but both understood the reason for her telling it. This was a bitter illustration, no doubt, but the two were able to glean from it the reassurance that they had been missing. Death was hard; they were watching it unfold. *But what they were seeing was not what their father was experiencing.* He apparently had a place to go, people to see, and a body that knew the way to get him there. With this realization, these two were able to cross another threshold, believing that God was doing the part that they could not. And the peace of the patient, rather than the effort to stop time, became the next cornerstone.

An Easy Death

Henry's mind and body continued to fade, and ten months after his admission to hospice, Henry left them. His breathing changed suddenly one afternoon, and three days later, he was gone. Lynette, who stayed with Daniel by the bedside during this period, updated the others often, notifying them of every period of wakefulness or mumbled word that he spoke. But the episodes had been brief, Henry falling back into a semiconsciousness that would remain again for hours.

On his last night, however, while Daniel was napping, Henry awoke, fully alert, and asked for a glass of milk—his first clear words in days. Lynette ran to the kitchen and returned quickly with the cold milk but found that her father was gone. It had happened just that quickly. She had been at her post for three days and nights, but somehow the last moment had been missed.

An Uneasy Bereavement

The funeral went well, the family members having had ample time to prepare. They then entered a new phase of grieving. The hospice bereavement counselor connected often, noticing that the one daughter was having more difficulty than the others with their father's passing. After several visits, Lynette was finally able to share her feelings with the counselor. She admitted that she felt betrayed and angry, feelings she knew were unfounded but ones she could not seem to shake. She had been the trustworthy one, the constant one, and yet her father had sneaked off behind her back. The hospice counselor, experienced in the unique emotions stirred by deathbed vigils, introduced a new interpretation of the event, hoping that perhaps this daughter would be able to switch an old belief for a new one and would be able to move on.

"You were also the safe one," the counselor gently reassured her. "And while the timing of your father's leaving may seem suspicious to you, I must tell you that it is more common than you would think—too common to be coincidental, in my experience. There seems to be an arrangement, almost a privacy pact of sorts, between the dying and the next world. I don't know what it is, but I have seen it enough times to make note of it." She related several other stories of family members she had known who sat by the side of their loved ones for years, only to go fill their coffee cup and return to find their loved one departed.

The bereavement counseling continued for several months more, and Lynette eventually allowed a reconciliation with her departed father. It came when she walked through the event once again with the counselor, this time seeing it through the eyes of her father. Was it possible that her father had been given no choice in the timing? Or that he had simply been allowed at just *that* moment to walk into the arms of his wife, his friends, his God—and had been purely and simply overcome by the experience as they ushered him away. "He's in a better place" had been proffered too many times in the past months and the words had cut bitterly, as if no one understood how she wanted him here, not there. But comfort was able to pierce through this day, and as she dropped a portion of her pain, she perceived a promise and a glimpse of hope for a second journey for Henry.

> If you can believe in what *could* be true;
> when your heart releases enough to remember
> what is promised and what is known
> rather than what is seen,
> then your grief becomes one step lifted.
>
> This has been a full-time but temporary job,
> and it is now a full-time but temporary loss.

You will never be the same, but could
this be a misplaced sadness?

If you can resolve to take the best parts of your loved one
and embed them into your own soul,
this recreated you, this new intertwining
will, in its time, pull you upwards.
Out of your grief and back into life,
your loved one becomes a deeper and closer part of and with you.
We never die, who have been loved.
—A.L.C.

Mr. Henry L. Sherman, aged seventy-six, passed away peacefully at his home, hospice bereavement services to follow.

QUESTIONS FOR REFLECTION
CHAPTER 1: HENRY

1. At some point in our lives, our personal desire to maintain our current condition is not able to overcome our physical limitations. Did you sense that Henry's heart failure was the creeping cause of his fatigue, or do you believe that his lack of interest in life was related to general depression caused by the loss of his wife and his former busy life?

2. A "Certificate of Terminal Illness" from a physician is required to qualify a patient for hospice services. Hospice is for the terminally ill rather than the chronically ill, and making this determination can be difficult. Some physicians are also reticent to discontinue treatments and procedures because of their professional commitment to save and extend life. Do you have a personal belief about when or if treatments should be discontinued?

3. No one in Henry's family knew what they were getting into when they decided to care for their father in his home rather than using the services of a nursing home. Daniel is the most available, but he is the least prepared for the tasks at hand. Some siblings may have found his approach to the diaper situation to be silly or demeaning to their father, but no one else was willing to take on the task. How do you feel about this? How might you have approached the situation?

4. A parent's illness is often the first time that adult siblings must come together to discuss major family decisions. Old sibling rivalries often obscure and overshadow the conversations. New relationships and new conversations require new skills. Mercy and patience are needed, yet it is crisis time. What reminders can you tell yourself when a conversation with your family is becoming tense? What gentle reminder can you speak out loud to your family when a conversation starts to "go south"?

5. Should your family open the discussion of the health and welfare of an aging parent now, rather than waiting until crisis time? Remembering that you will all grow older and may need help from each other, are there current relationships with siblings that need mending, and can you be the first to reach out?

CHAPTER 2

Tracy's Journey

- Age 51
- Chronic obstructive pulmonary disease (COPD)
- Primary symptom: respiratory failure
- Primary caregiver: Tabitha (54)

The Road Together

Trainwreck Tracy

Tracy Moore is a fifty-one-year-old female with a long history of drug addiction. She lives in a small house on a back road, forty miles from any large city. Tracy is in the end stages of COPD, a respiratory disease most likely brought on by years of smoking and complicated by drug use. Tracy lives alone but has a community of friends, some good, some not so good. They drive her to doctor appointments, bring her groceries, lend her money, and then borrow it back. The borrowing is not always repaid, and the recompense is not always balanced. Tracy lives in the system behind the system—a loose cooperative with its own values and rules. There are common themes and bylaws understood by all, and Tracy maneuvers them as well as any stockbroker on Wall Street does the markets.

Tracy is a frequent flyer in the local emergency room, and her hospital chart is several inches thick, earning her the nickname of "Trainwreck Tracy." Every few months, Tracy barges through the double doors, grungy, twitchy, and out of control, her chest heaving, her face panic-stricken. Her frenzy in the waiting room snags her a jump to the head of the line, and she is rushed back for a barrage of rescue inhalers and breathing treatments. Sometimes, she is discharged home with a prescription of opioids for her symptoms, sometimes not. Anyone observing the distress of the emaciated woman would have compassion on her. Her shoulders heave, her ribs retract, and her face is drawn and ashen; her x-rays confirm lungs filled with solidified congestion. But now the prescribed medications don't seem to help, and her opioid medications are gone within a few days. The revolving door that earned her the nickname and the reputation is closing—Tracy is dying.

Tracy and Hospice

Tracy is used to dying. She has been admitted to hospice four times to date, her clinical reports and physical exam qualifying her every time. Each time hospice care is initiated, Tracy immediately improves. Her medications are regulated, and her home-delivered meals are reinstated. She receives an aide to give her a good bath, and she is encouraged by the friendly visits. Her family also receives regular updates, which increases their involvement in Tracy's life.

But then Tracy falls off the wagon. Her medications disappear, and she can't be found for the mandatory minimal visits. Her home meals pile up outside her door. The hospice agency is eventually forced to discharge for noncompliance, and the family throws up their hands again in frustration. Tracy doesn't want to live life in the main system—it's restrictive, and there are too many rules. But life behind the system has also taken its toll, and Tracy has burned bridges in both.

The emergency room physician knows Tracy well. He has tracked the progression of her disease for years. He has marked the steady weight loss, the thickening of her chest and the clubbing of her fingers, the sallowness of her complexion, and the fear in her eyes. He also understands that this is why she frequents his ER. Despite her scrawny toughness, Tracy Moore is afraid.

Tracy and Tabitha

When Tracy's name appeared on the intake roster, the staff braced for mayhem. Tracy's final entrance was not the usual, however. She sat still and small in the rear of the waiting room, her weight loss alarming to those who knew her. And most unusual was that she was in the company of her older sister. Their relationship was known to be a strained one.

Tracy was fully coherent this visit but was notably weak. She reported that she had been in bed for two weeks, nauseated and lethargic and unable to eat. She required help to transfer from the wheelchair to the exam table. Her oxygen levels were low, and they improved little with treatments. Her x-rays were unchanged from her last visit a few months ago—still terrible. Tracy was admitted to the hospital but was little improved when she was discharged three days later. She was able to walk to the bathroom with help, but her appetite remained poor and her breathing continued labored. It was agreed that Tracy would be discharged to her sister's care with hospice to follow.

Tabitha, along with her daughter, Carrie, lived in a quaint three-bedroom house in the center of town. Tabitha began laying down the law as she drove Tracy home—no visitors, no drugs, no smoking in the house. Act civilly, and you'll be allowed to stay. Tracy had little choice but to agree; she was too weak and had no breath for arguing. She simply nodded an unenthused "yes" to each of Tabitha's demands.

Tabitha worked as the night shift manager at the local grocery, and Carrie worked the baked goods counter, which meant that the enticing smells of doughnuts and fresh baked bread often lingered on her when she left work. Tracy loved this about her niece, and she was known to hang on a few extra moments whenever she had the opportunity to hug her. But this time, as Carrie leaned into the car to help lift Tracy out, a wave of nausea swept over Tracy, and she begged to be released. So it was her sister who assisted Tracy up the stairs and into the house as Carrie followed. The question crossing each mind in that moment was whether Tracy would ever walk back down these steps again.

Tracy was grateful to finally lie down in the hospital bed, which had been delivered that morning. She longed for a marijuana cigarette to combat the nausea, but she hadn't any left. She supposed that she would have to resort to the prescription medications and suffer their side effects. Stray thoughts occupied her mind as she lay back on the pillow, staring up at Tabitha's painted ceiling. The hospital admission, the displacement of finding herself at her sister's house, the replay of hospice ... she couldn't help but wonder if she would be able to surprise death again, or would her luck run out this time? It was hours before she was finally able to rest.

Tracy's Addictive Past

Hospice made their admission visit the next day, though they knew Tracy Moore well. The assessment confirmed that Tracy had indeed declined and that she once again qualified for their services. The nurse and aide visits were scheduled, as well as social worker and chaplain visits. Tabitha also requested a few hours of volunteer services each week in order to keep her own counselor appointments. Growing up had not been easy for these two sisters.

Tabitha listened in as Tracy catalogued her symptoms to the nurse. Pain, anxiety, nausea, cough, unable to take a deep breath in, unable to push air back out, sleeplessness, headaches, numbness and pain in her legs, a knot in her stomach, dry mouth from the oxygen—pretty much everything was either hurting or not working. Tracy did not have to look over to see the familiar eye roll of her sister, but it was important to her that the nurse order all the appropriate medications, since she would have no access to the remedies she preferred.

With the assessment completed, Tabitha escorted the nurse out of Tracy's room, pulling the door closed behind them. As the latch caught, Tracy was reaching for the bottle of

> Hospice and the addict

anxiety pills from the hospital. She swallowed one and then two more. It had been a long day, and it was still morning.

On the other side of the latch, Tabitha was cornering the nurse.

"I don't want my sister overmedicated in this house," she announced. "We filled the hospital prescriptions on the way home, and when they're gone, that's it. I don't want anything stronger than an aspirin for her. I know that she's faking; it's the way she works. And I don't want my daughter influenced by all of this. It's hard enough just having Tracy here. We tried this once before, and it did not work. She smoked pot, she burned my couch with cigarette ashes, she'd pass out on the floor from who knows what. She's been on hospice before too, and they just give her more drugs—why do you do that? She's an addict! Why would you give her drugs?" Tabitha had been holding on to this question for quite some time, and it came out harsher than she had intended. But she had not slept well, staying in Tracy's room at the hospital, and she was tired before they even got started. She stood with her arms crossed tightly against her chest, her vexation poorly contained. The nurse motioned her over to the couch, moving her further away from Tracy's room. Tracy was having enough difficulty without taking on others' moods.

As they crossed the room, the nurse reminded herself that this was not a personal challenge toward her nor toward her agency; this was simply a person who had been hurt many times over and needed to vent. It was not unusual for families to find themselves unexpectedly thrown together by illness but still experiencing unresolved issues from their pasts. She hoped they would be able to help the sisters find new ground, *if* Tracy was still able to participate.

"I hear your frustration." The nurse nodded with understanding. "We are frustrated as well at times. The hospice goal is to provide comfort and dignity through the end of life. This gets difficult when a person can't or won't follow the plan of care. But there are guidelines in place that help us manage the pain and anxiety that is often driving the abuse." Tabitha looked at her warily, but the nurse continued, undaunted. She went on to reassure Tabitha that the hospice physician was very familiar with substance abuse and end-stage diseases and that the team would work together to find the right medications and doses that would provide relief for Tracy but would not promote her addiction.

"She's still going to call the ambulance when she feels bad," Tabitha rebutted, holding her ground. But her arms were loosening their tight grip.

"People aren't always thinking things through, are they?" The nurse sighed, granting the possibility. "The hospital told her that there was nothing else they could do for her, and we will remind Tracy that insurance doesn't pay for medical services in her home and also at the hospital that are related to her terminal diagnosis. She might receive a bill from the hospital, or she may be discharged from hospice, or both things may happen. Our agency's hope and goal, though, is to provide Tracy with the medication balance at home that she needs. We want her to call us, rather than calling 911. And, Tabitha, things do look different this time. Perhaps this is the time she'll let us help her."

Tabitha agreed that her sister's condition did appear to be direr than any time before, but she also knew Tracy much better than this nurse did. Tracy could be tricky.

> "Call us before calling 911."

Is She Truly Sick?

"So you're thinking she might not be faking this time?" Little sister had been "sick" a long time.

"I believe that Tracy is very uncomfortable right now," the nurse affirmed. "It takes considerable muscle work for her to pull in only a small breath of air and then push it back out again. It can make sitting in a chair feel like jogging up a mountain. You and I aren't familiar with this fatigue, but a COPD patient is. And since Tracy can't breathe well, she doesn't move around much. This causes muscles and joints to stiffen and ache. Her low oxygen levels create headaches and more body weakness. And, of course, there are the immediate symptoms of anxiousness, and an unnamed fear that comes when the body is not able to get the level of oxygen that it craves."

The nurse stopped, giving Tabitha time for review, hoping that she would allow that at least some of Tracy's complaints might be justified. But Tabitha was forecasting on a different level. If she agreed that Tracy was in pain, then she would have to allow narcotics and whatever else to come into her home, and this would be a game changer if Tracy pulled her usual tricks. But she was also seeing for herself the difference in Tracy's mood and energy. She supposed she should at least hear the nurse out.

"So what's your plan then?" she exhaled guardedly.

The nurse had her mini-lesson prepared and scooted to the edge of the couch.

Hospice Medications and the Addict

"I know that you are concerned about Tracy's addiction history, so let me start there. Addiction occurs when you take more pain medication than the level of pain that you are experiencing. Most drug abusers have no pain when they take a drug; therefore, they feel a high. But if you take an appropriate dose for your pain, then you have no high and you function better in your day. Let me give you an example: if you were to break your ankle and were going in to physical therapy, you would take your pain pill first, correct? Not so much that you can't function but enough for you to be effective in your workout."

Tabitha interrupted her. "But she isn't going to therapy; she's just lying in bed."

The nurse countered. "For some, simply turning over in bed can feel like a therapy workout." Tabitha began an eye roll but caught herself. She was trying. The nurse noticed and gave her a quick smile before continuing on.

> Addiction and comfort medications

"We use several types of meds to meet our patient's needs, and we will teach you how to administer them. The medications will address three types of pain: maintenance, breakthrough, and immediate need. The philosophy is not to 'knock them out' with medications but also for your loved one to not be knocked out by their pain. Try not to be overly concerned at this point, Tabitha. We will walk you through it as many times as you need, until you are comfortable."

But Tabitha had become very concerned. She would be giving Tracy her medicines? She hadn't thought about that. The nurse paused, familiar with the struggle. The topic of medications and their administration often prompted more apprehension than reassurance in families, swiftly hauling the caregiver out of good intentions and into stark reality. Tabitha was overcome by the idea of handing out medications to her addict sister, even if she *was* that sick. Her arms tightened around her chest again, her eyes closing tightly over a difficult situation that just got worse.

The Plan Is Good, Even If the Path Is Hard

Tabitha's eyes finally opened, and she turned to face the nurse. Her expression confessed every emotion that she had been holding in restraint, ever since the phone call four days ago when Tracy had asked for a ride to the emergency room. An old and endless conflict was filling up inside her. She got to her feet without warning, striding over to stand at Tracy's closed door. She did not open it but just stood before it, staring into the white emptiness of the woodwork. The nurse remained quiet, knowing that the emotions behind caregiving were even more important than the actual giving of the care itself. It never worked when a caregiver was coerced into this role. She thought back to her own personal and professional hopes for this family—peace and comfort for Tracy and reconciliation and a clear conscience for Tabitha. Adjustments between head and heart required time, and Tabitha was deeply submersed in an internal renegotiation. Should she continue with this crazy idea of taking care of her crazy sister, or should she turn Tracy back out to the streets as good sense dictated? It was a weighty decision, and the nurse remained patient while Tabitha stared desperately, contemplating the choice. The intention of the plan was good, but this path would be hard.

When Tabitha finally pivoted and returned to the couch, her disheartened walk spilled out the decision. Gone was her anger and, with it, her energy. She would not be throwing Tracy out. Tears pooled in her eyes, and her voice was weary when she spoke.

"I just don't know how I'm going to manage this," she whispered, her shoulders slumping forward in surrender, her palms open, asking.

Tabitha's Choice

They sat quietly for a moment, considering. The nurse was more aware than Tabitha of the hardships that would come in the next days and weeks. Yes, the nurse thought, this choice carried with it a heavy burden. There was nothing to be added at the moment to encourage Tabitha, as they both knew that the bulk of the burden would fall to her. So the nurse decided to build on the love that had originally prompted her to invite her sister back into her life.

> *You don't choose hospice; hospice chooses you.*

"We all just do the best that we can, Tabitha. It becomes difficult sometimes, and the answers are not always clear. But we continue to try. Thank you for loving your sister enough to stand in this gap with her. We can only pray that someone will do it for us when it's our turn."

Tabitha's tears spilled in earnest now. The nurse was right. She was afraid of what was to come, but she did love her sister and did not want her to be alone—especially now, if this was truly her end. The nurse waited again until the wave of emotion ebbed and Tabitha recovered, dabbing her eyes with her sleeve. She looked up and engaged the nurse for one last round regarding the dreaded medications.

"Tracy's not going to let me keep her medicines," she said, resignedly. "I'm sure of that. So how will we manage them?"

The nurse returned to the theme, relieved that Tabitha was still in Tracy's game.

"The lines are obscured sometimes," she admitted honestly. "If a patient is in their full mind, then they have the right to manage their own medicines. Maybe Tracy will agree to a medicine planner and will let you keep the rest of her meds locked away. We will be clear with her that if she runs out of medications early, they will not be refilled until the next due date. But we hold the belief that everybody gets a chance to try it. I have found that addicts tend to be very savvy about their meds. They know how to parcel them out to cover their needs. Again, my hope is that this is the time that Tracy will be compliant."

Tabitha shrugged a noncommittal maybe. She had tired again and had no more energy to give the topic. They talked over a few last details, and the nurse closed her visit. As she rose to leave, Tabitha placed a hand on her arm with one last burning question. She hesitated before speaking. "I know this sounds morbid, but I need to plan. How long do you think she has?" Tabitha's question was direct, but it was not an unfamiliar one for the hospice nurse. She eased back down to her seat.

How Long Does She Have?

"We never know, of course, and when I hazard to guess, I'm usually wrong. I can tell you that she seems to have slipped a significant level even in the past week, according to her chart. The hospital was not able to find anything to account for her sudden weakness, so they believe it to be the progression of her disease.

> Saw-tooth pattern

Many illnesses often follow a 'saw-tooth' pattern of decline, which looks like, well, a handsaw that is tilted down on one end. There is a gradual decline, punctuated by episodes of severe illness. The patient recovers from the episodes, but not fully. Each episode takes a little more out of them, until they are at their last episode. We will have to wait and see if this is the final flare and Tracy has days to weeks, or, hopefully, she will get a little better and will have weeks to months."

Tabitha nodded her understanding. This pattern of sickness and rebound was familiar.

The nurse rose again, pulling her equipment bag to her shoulder. "I'll set up a return visit for tomorrow. Is there anything else that I can do for you?" Tabitha shook her head no. She had much to contemplate as it was.

She walked the nurse to the front door and then returned to Tracy's room, opening the door quietly. Tracy was curled on her side, facing the wall. The oxygen concentrator was loud in the room, but Tracy had heard the door and rolled over as her sister entered.

How Bad Am I?

"How do you feel about the nurse visit?" Tabitha offered hesitantly, aware that Tracy may have overheard her tirade. She pulled a chair close to the bed.

"I'm afraid," Tracy answered, faltering. She had heard, but she had deeper worries of her own. "I'm trying not to be, but I am. I think that I've been trying to die all of my life, Tabby, but now that it's here, I want to take it all back. I'm not ready to die yet."

Tabitha's mouth began to form her conditioned response of "This is what you get," but she stopped herself. Tracy looked so frail in the hospital bed, and the reciprocal antagonism and fire in her eyes was absent. Tabitha thought she looked more like the little sister who had hidden herself under the covers when their father had one of his rages—before she had determined to fight back. Tracy had been fighting life ever since. No wonder she was tired. And hadn't the nurse said that fear was a natural part of this disease? Maybe her little sister had been the stronger one after all.

"Would you like me to turn your oxygen up? Or get you some water? Carrie has mom's spaghetti recipe on the stove. It's your favorite. You'll feel better when you eat something."

Tracy looked a little nauseous at the mention of food.

"I'll try," she said blandly, "but food tastes like cardboard to me somehow. I think about food all the time, but it's like my mouth has forgotten how to eat it."

She was quiet after that, and they sat in silence. Conversation had always been difficult between them. Their last years had contained only battles and arguments. Tracy borrowed money and didn't pay it back. Tracy had wrecked Tabitha's car. Tracy was in jail again. Tabitha realized that she had simply not known what to do with her little sister. She wanted to love her, but Tracy had not let her in.

"Tell me what the nurse said," Tracy interjected into her thoughts. "Tell me what's going to happen to me. Don't hold back." Her eyes found Tabitha's, reading her face. What should she say?

"Well," Tabitha started slowly, "she said that you look good and that she is glad that you are staying with me. They are going to put you on some medicines to help you with your pain and your breathing." Then she took the opportunity and spilled out her greatest worry.

"The nurse did tell me that if you run out of medicines early, they can't be refilled, Tracy. You'll just have to stick it out. Do you understand that? And she suggested a pill planner so that you don't get confused." Tabitha decided not to mention the lockbox she was planning to buy.

Talking with your loved one

"Did she say that I'm dying?" Tracy sidestepped, a more important concern on her mind.

It was Tabitha who looked away first.

"She didn't say, Tracy. She explained that your COPD has

episodes of sickness that you bounce back from, but each time that you get sick, you become a little weaker. She said we'd have to wait and see."

"I don't feel like I'm bouncing back from this one at all," Tracy murmured, her gaze dropping to the bedrail between them. "I feel so weak this time, like my body wants to fall into the deepest sleep ever. But every time my eyes close, I jerk awake in a panic. I know there's nothing they can do to make my lungs better. All they can do is just give me more medicines. But they don't work, Tabitha. Even the marijuana doesn't relax me enough to make me feel safe. I feel like I'm losing my grip, and I'm just going to slide off a mountain or something. All I can think about is staying awake so that I don't die in my sleep." She blinked her eyes, tears pooling but not falling. She couldn't afford to cry; it required too much air. "I don't want to die," she said again, closing her eyes.

Tabitha didn't know what to say. She had compassion but still felt the intermix of older feelings. She'd seen her sister play the victim card so often. But what if things were true this time? What if her sister was to actually die?

Tabitha leaned over to kiss Tracy on the forehead and then walked briskly out of the room, overcome, but in a different way now. She was still fighting her inner battle but was surprised to find a new determination forming. Arising from the old resolve against her sister, there appeared a new resolve *for* her sister, a desire to protect her like she had when they were young. Tabitha made a sudden and surprisingly solid decision for herself. She would stand by her sister. It no longer mattered whether Tracy deserved it or not. This was something that she would do for herself *and* for her sister, so that there would be no bad blood between them. She wanted no regrets for either of them when Tracy left this world. If that meant losing work, staying up all hours, listening to Tracy whine, or even wiping Tracy's backside, Tabitha would do it for her own higher reasons. She hoped that the snippets of compassion that whisked in and out of her would grow to overpower the past hurts. There was so much to forgive here, on both sides. She prayed that they would have enough time to repair things, even if just a little. As the nurse had said, everybody deserves compassion and dignity at the end of their life. Tabitha determined to claim this blessing for herself as well.

The Path Bends

Two weeks passed in the small house, but Tracy showed no improvement. Tabitha's predictions of medication struggles turned out to be mostly unfounded, not because Tracy had suddenly become compliant, but because she had lost energy for the battle. The pills from the hospital had disappeared quickly, but since then, Tracy had given Tabitha the steering wheel. The narcotics were carefully titrated by the nurse, and doses had indeed been found that helped Tracy's discomfort but did not oversedate her. She requested her breakthrough medications more frequently than Tabitha judged necessary, but accepting that only the prescribed number of pills was available, Tracy kept to the schedule. And for the most part, she found her fears and symptoms contained.

The Crossroads

Transition

The third week was similar with one marked exception. Tracy refused to eat. Maybe a bite here or there at Carrie or Tabitha's insistence but not enough to sustain life. Tabitha was waiting at the door when the nurse arrived.

"She's getting weaker because she won't eat. Are we just going to let her starve?" Tabitha looked frayed around the edges, but her tone was strong and insistent. She had taken her charge very seriously, and Tracy's welfare to the very end was her newfound mission. "There's got to be something to do. Can she get a feeding tube? What do you do for people who won't eat?"

The nurse had become accustomed to Tabitha's doorway barrages, but her heart dropped now for this sister who had finally found a way to love the prodigal. She knew that sudden loss of appetite was a part of the dying process, and there would be no stopping it. The rising chemicals in the body turned the digestive switches off so that it could attend to the more important matters of filling the lungs and pumping the heart. Tracy was nearing her final weeks. The nurse chose her next words carefully, kindly.

"If a person can't eat," she began while slipping off her jacket, "a doctor may consider putting a feeding tube into the stomach, though this is rarely suggested in hospice. But first we have to determine *why* the person cannot eat. It sounds like Tracy may be entering a phase we call transition. It basically means a change of direction."

> End-of-life and feeding tubes

"Go on. I'm listening." Tabitha's arms had crossed. Not a good sign.

"Let's sit down, and I'll draw the process out for you; then you can decide for yourself." In the nurse's experience, the family's mind already knew what their hearts could not yet accept.

They sat down, Tabitha's arms wrapped tightly around her middle. The nurse spoke slowly and clearly, as if breaking the news to a family in the emergency room that their loved one was not going to pull through. It crossed her mind briefly to ask once again why she chose this job, but as she recalled her own life stories, she knew. You don't choose hospice; hospice chooses you. She took a breath and turned to face Tabitha.

"There are several organ systems in the body. The two main systems are the heart and the lungs. When either of these shuts down, the body immediately fails. When there are not enough resources to keep all of the systems going, the body begins shutting down the less important organs first. It often begins with the digestive system. I know that eating sounds very important, but

A Journey of One 35

it takes a lot of internal energy to digest food, and when you are down to the last choice of a stomach or a heart, the body chooses the heart. Tracy is not eating because her body cannot spare the energy anymore."

The nurse looked at Tabitha, who appeared to be disappointed by this response but not crestfallen. The answer was not too much of a surprise.

"So how long does this transition phase last?" Tabitha asked, resignation in her voice.

"People are different," the nurse said carefully, counting her words. "But in my experience, death usually occurs two to four weeks after a person stops eating. But, Tabitha, it could also be just a few days. We really can't predict these things." Tabitha caught her breath. She appreciated the candor, but things were apparently as bad as she feared.

The nurse left to make her assessment with Tracy and then came back to sit. But her opinion had not changed. She spent the remainder of the visit educating Tabitha on the symptoms to anticipate during the next course and she jotted down a new medication schedule. She also increased the staffing visits to ensure that both Tracy and Tabitha were comfortable with the coming changes. She left then, and Tabitha went to sit in Tracy's room, the conversations and silences no longer uncomfortable. All they had needed was a little practice.

- Decline
- Transition
- Actively dying

Near the end of the fourth week, it was Carrie who called the hospice office. Tracy had woken up gasping, and her breathing was very rapid and shallow. The house was in a panic. The medications were not calming her, and they didn't know what else to do. The nurse in the office spoke reassuringly to Carrie, instructing her to turn up the oxygen and for Tabitha to administer a dose of the emergency medication that was on hand. She scheduled an urgent visit for Tracy, and a nurse was sent out to help.

A Journey of One

Actively Dying

Tracy was little changed when the nurse arrived. Her pulse was weak and thready, and her blood pressure and oxygen levels were too low to be measured. Tracy's temperature had risen to 104°, which the nurse said was not unusual in the end stages. The nurse administered a combination of medications from the lockbox and then placed a call to the doctor for further orders. Tracy was confused and anxious, sitting up in the bed, her eyes wide, then falling back limply against the pillows, breathless. Tabitha felt great relief that the nurse was present—this was a bit more frightening than she had counted on, and she was feeling helpless in it. Once the nurse arrived, Carrie left for a friend's house, and Tabitha was grateful to not have the worry of both daughter and sister that day.

When it was obvious that she could do nothing else to help, Tabitha climbed into the bed with Tracy, squeezing behind her to support her back. She felt her little sister immediately relax against her, her head lolling against Tabitha's shoulder. She kissed the top of Tracy's head softly. Tracy couldn't cry, so Tabitha cried for both of them, silently, so as not to add to the distress of her exhausted sister. The medicine from the lockbox took another hour to work, but soon Tracy was resting comfortably, leaning heavily into her sister's arms. Her pulse and breathing remained shallow; her oxygen levels did not rise. The nurse prepared Tabitha that Tracy appeared to be approaching her end. She called the office and arranged for continuous care staffing, reassuring Tabitha that she would not be left alone. Tracy roused again only a handful of times during the long day, wild-eyed and gasping, until a therapeutic medication level was regained. The day turned into evening, and a depleted Tracy was resting calmly again. Occasionally, her eyes would flutter open, and a light squeeze would pulse Tabitha's hand, making sure big sister was still there. The connections were brief, and Tracy, reassured, tumbled back into heavy sleep.

Tracy Moore took her last breath in the early morning, just before sunrise. Tabitha was dozing, cramped up in the hospital bed, but still holding her sister against her chest. She woke as she felt Tracy's chest rising sharply. There was one deep breath in and then a long, last breath out. There were no more. The reconciliation was complete, and the sisters' paths divided once more.

Tracy Moore, aged fifty-one, passed away peacefully at the home of her sister, hospice bereavement services to follow.

QUESTIONS FOR REFLECTION
CHAPTER 2: TRACY

1. The relationship between Tracy and Tabitha had always been rocky, and now Tracy requires help once again. Do you have a family member who can't seem to get his or her life together and comes to you often for help? Have you ever been that family member? How did you relate to Tabitha and her difficult decision?

2. Medications and illness are always hot topics. Should the doctors give more or give less? Should the patient take everything that a doctor prescribes? How are the side effects affecting the patient? The family? How would you feel about hospice medications being brought into your home?

3. When Tracy asks Tabitha about her condition, Tabitha is unsure of how to reply. Many times, telling the truth brings fear, but sometimes it brings peace because the family is finally talking about things. Each conversation demands kindness and simplicity and must allow for all members to roam in and out of the stages of grief (denial, anger, bargaining, depression, acceptance) without fear of judgment. What do you feel when you see that someone is in denial about his or her condition? What do you feel when the person's worsening condition affects you too?

4. What are your feelings about Tabitha's daughter, Carrie? She would have grown up with family encounters of "Trainwreck Tracy." Should she have been present for her aunt's death, or are you glad that she left for a friend's house? What do you feel about younger children being present for a death?

5. Loss of appetite is often the first real sign that the end is approaching, and our first tendency is to do everything possible to correct this situation. Do you have personal experience with someone who has been given a feeding tube? Do you feel that it had a positive or a negative outcome? Do you want a feeding tube for yourself, and have you made known your own living will preferences?

CHAPTER 3

Jon's Journey

- Age 88, Alzheimer's disease
- Primary symptom: dementia
- Caregiver: Maggie (78)

The Road Together

Jon and Maggie

Jonas "Jon" MacDouglas is an eighty-eight-year-old male with a terminal diagnosis of end-stage Alzheimer's dementia. Diagnosed seven years ago, it started as the usual—forgetting words, misplacing items, losing his car in the parking lot, unclear of days and dates. There was little concern at first; after all, he was eighty-one and wasn't old age wonderful, that you were no longer expected to keep up with the details of life? Jon voluntarily relinquished his driver's license two years following his diagnosis when he became confused in a grocery store, requiring his wife to come get him. Entering the store, she saw her husband handing the grocer his open wallet. It was then she realized that she was soon to become not only the keeper of the car and the money but of her husband as well.

Jon and his wife, Maggie, ten years his junior, still lived in their original home of sixty-two years. Their only child lived several states away, his wife having pressed him to move closer to her family. The two of them returned home every Christmas until, in his forties, their son was diagnosed with Parkinson's disease and was soon unable to travel. Even then, he still called regularly until the Parkinson's took him at age fifty. He had been a good son. His wife? Well, it was best to not talk about that.

Jon towered above Maggie's five-foot frame, but that petite frame contained the spirit of a heavyweight prizefighter. Jon's memory might be slipping, but he never forgot who was the boss. Maggie kept a sharp eye on him. Because of her vigilance, they had been able to sidestep many of the accidents and pitfalls that other dementia sufferers often experienced. Early in his diagnosis, Maggie had promised to keep Jon safe, happy, and at home, and she now dedicated her days to this end.

Jon MacDouglas had been a structured man who trusted in self-sufficiency and routine. He wore a suit and tie every day to work, cut the grass on Saturday, and expected his dinners at 6:00 p.m. every evening. His orderly manner had made for a simple married life, which suited Maggie fine, having been raised in the chaotic home of a mentally ill mother. Jon and Maggie were both wary of what the world had to offer, and that had served to bond them tightly together against it.

Maggie ran a tight ship: "a place for everything and everything in its place." Conversation was frugal, remanded to the basics of household concerns—where had Maggie laid Jon's glasses, when was Jon going to get around to the leaky faucet. The television was rarely on, the news only reinforcing their desire to stay clear of "the craziness in the world." Both were comfortable in their quietness, Jon snoozing contentedly in front of an old western after supper and Maggie working on her latest needlepoint project until bedtime.

Losing Him before She Lost Him

But that was "before Alzheimer's." This new companion—one that resembled her husband but contained only the odds and ends of him—was a shadow, a mimicry of sorts. This fellow was almost a doppelganger, being the active opposite of the Jon she knew. He didn't sit, he didn't snooze, he couldn't focus on a movie, and for some reason, he wouldn't leave her house alone. Her Jon had never cared where things were before, because Maggie simply brought what he needed to him. But by some trick of flickering synapses, this Jon was convinced that he was the newly self-appointed superintendent of the home. He would randomly launch from his chair, moving determinedly to cabinets and closets, pulling out towels and folded clothes, emptying entire drawers onto the floor, switching the bread with the toilet paper and the ketchup for the shampoo. There was no stopping him when he was in his "go mode." Jon was a tall, lean, self-possessed man on a mission.

> Adjusting to dementia

Besides the rummaging and reorganizing, Jon would also compulsively (and slyly, to Maggie's incredulity) leave the house. She heard the car start one morning and ran to find Jon sitting in the front seat, boxers loose on his thinning hips, heading to work. That scare initiated the installation of key pads and locks on all the doors, and more household adaptations were to follow. But Jon could solve any child lock, so Maggie was obliged to empty out her cabinet shelves and ransom only her pantry, securing it with a deadbolt and keeping the key around her neck. She left the refrigerator door unhindered, however, as Jon's favorite activity was to "clean out the fridge." His overambitious mind needed entertaining, and this enterprise seemed to provide him with a sense of accomplishment as well. After relocating all the items to the countertops and the floor, he would stand back, hands cocked on his hips, beaming into the empty box. Maggie added the repacking of the refrigerator to her nightly routine, once she was sure that Jon had fallen asleep.

When the circadian clock of Jon's brain stopped ticking and he no longer responded to daytime and nighttime cues, Maggie accommodated. She tied a bell to the doorknob and slept on the side of the bed closest to the door. She was up in a flash when she heard the jingle, surreptitiously shadowing Jon as he padded to the bathroom or down the hallway, maybe shuffling to play the refrigerator game again or sometimes just to stare at the padlock on the basement door that led down to his forgotten workshop.

Early Dementia

During the early years, Maggie tried reorienting her muddled husband.

"It's nighttime, Jon. Come back to bed," or "You've had supper already, Jon. Please get out of the refrigerator." But she finally gave way, accepting that her corrections only caused anxiety for Jon, and they were creating a crushing resentment in her. Poor Jon couldn't grasp her admonitions; he sensed only that he was out of step in some way. Odd thing, to have no real communication or processing skills but to still retain self-consciousness and shame. In grace for them both, Maggie refrained from her compulsion to set things right. She began new conversations with Jon, reminiscing and speaking kindnesses—entering his world and his pace. She carried on their disjointed relationship as best she could, knowing that she surely sounded as crazy as he did, but doing what she could to fend off the edges of unfamiliar loneliness.

> Beyond reorientation

As the tedious years continued, Jon lost muscle mass, and his already long face took on an angular and wide-eyed countenance. Maggie was showing physical signs of strain as well. She experienced dizzy spells, and her ankles were swollen. But who had time to go to the doctor! As it was, Maggie risked only a few minutes for a quick grocery or errand run, praying that Jon would stay put in his recliner. If a more extensive excursion was required, Maggie reluctantly asked a neighbor for help. Whether they were disinclined on their own or whether Maggie read into it she couldn't tell, but the exchanges were always uncomfortable. Maggie supposed her neighbors were worried that they would become responsible for this quirky, solitary couple, and Maggie could not blame them. But it was best if she did not think about it too much, and she solicited help only when absolutely necessary.

The Path Bends

Maggie fared well enough with the unending disruption of her home, Jon's wandering, and her sleep deprivation, but bath time had begun to wipe her out. They had been such an adorable couple in their early years, his handsome face bending deeply to meet hers, her diminutive frame stretching high on tiptoe to receive his kiss. But now his cumbersome height was the straw that might break the camel's back—and hers. She simply could not make Jon understand that he had to bend his head much lower in order for her to shampoo him. And he was always walking away before she completed the rinsing or the toweling.

Then followed the ominous day when Jon misplaced the toilet. Maggie's scrupulous and modest husband now saw any potted plant, sink, or corner of the house as a potential urinal. Maggie's sharp mind hustled, trying everything she could imagine. She purchased all types of

> Adjusting again

adult diapers and pull-ups, but Jon refused to let her put them on him. If she was able to distract him and eventually slip one on, he simply yanked it down to take care of business. And, as was his new way, he often walked away before the task was complete. Maggie kept a Lysol bucket at the ready and cleaned the carpets regularly. She doubled the diapers, doubled the pants, and fastened a tight belt around his waist, but the problem was unsolvable. She finally surrendered and planned for a remodel when all this was over—if the Lord didn't take her first.

Milestones and Touchstones

These years took their toll, and Maggie was somewhat grateful that she had little time to think. She knew in the quiet corners of her mind that their lives were slipping away, and she was often aware of the somberness that lingered in the rooms with them, despite her efforts to keep it pushed back. She tried refocusing on the gift that her Jon was still here, though only a small part of him was truly recognizable to her. On good days, Jon was cheerful and chatty in his own unintelligible language, sometimes bringing her gifts, such as a button or a spoon, sometimes bursting into song, every lyric miraculously recited. Even on bad days, when Jon seemed to have forgotten her completely, they were still touchstones for each other. She would look up to see where he was and would catch him looking back, like two children seeking reassurance that they are not lost.

FAST Scale: Stage 7

Time passed, as did the unlacing of Jon's mind. The mad activity of the early years faded, and Maggie marked the slips and shifts—the longer periods of silence, the frequent naps. One particular morning as she sat at the kitchen table, weariness and sadness rising with her from her bed, Maggie allowed herself a rare moment of unreserved tears. She was losing Jon before she lost him. It felt as if they were peering together from inside a forest and all paths out had closed over. The thought made her sit up sharply, a sudden urge possessing her to understand more about this forest.

She brushed her tears away and tried to remember their last neurology appointment, when Jon had been officially labeled. Hadn't there been a packet or some papers from that day? Where could she have placed them? She deserted her cup of coffee to search the empty drawers of the kitchen and the living room and then crept quietly down the hall to the locked door of the office. She felt a bit like Jon, covertly compassing the house. But there was a shift in her now. She wondered at it briefly. A new energy fueled by ... anger? Fear? But she would know where this awful disease was leading them.

As she pulled open file cabinets and drawers, Maggie reviewed what she already knew of Alzheimer's. Her grandmother had passed away with something similar, but all she could remember was a sweet old lady nodding absently in her rocking chair. Jon's parents had both had their full minds intact when they had passed. There had been a few acquaintances diagnosed with the disease, but at some point, they had simply disappeared behind closed doors. Now, she realized, she was behind the door and didn't know what was ahead.

She finally found the blue folder, creased and bent, under a stack of old bills. She recognized the image of the well-coiffed man and woman standing in a garden, and she recalled the churning of her stomach when the nurse had handed it to her. The doctor was just stepping out, having delivered the bad news. Jon had been quiet that visit, contentedly sitting on the exam table while the doctor had talked to Maggie. "When Someone You Love Is Diagnosed with Alzheimer's Disease" the folder read. She returned to the kitchen, scanning the contents as she walked.

FAST scale for Alzheimer's dementia

The enclosed booklet was of a general nature, addressing the basics, of which Maggie was by now a crackerjack. She laid the booklet aside and flipped through the stack of handouts—"Agency Referrals," "Safety Tips," "The Caregiver's Role"—until she came to a chart labeled "FAST Scale: Functional Assessment Staging Tool for Alzheimer's Disease." Maggie vaguely remembered the nurse referring to this chart as a rule of thumb rather than a true directional chart, as symptoms advance differently in Alzheimer's sufferers. But Maggie became acutely aware, as she skimmed the chart, that Jon had indeed been working his way down the list. He was more than halfway through by now—much more than halfway. It was distressing, in fact, to see that Jon had hit all of the markers of Stages 1 through 6. And there were only 7 stages on the scale.

She cursorily surveyed Jon's past year in her mind. He had certainly been sleeping more, but she had been grateful for the extra rest and had registered it as progress rather than decline. The early indicators of stage 7 referred to a sufferer's loss of the ability to speak. Jon mumbled in his sleep every night, and he continued to ask his usual questions to no one in particular—where was his suit jacket, was his dad coming over today, was supper ready, and so on. But the house had definitely reclaimed its customary quietness. How had she not noticed this? She was devastated by this detail that now identified itself as a blazing landmark. Jon's constant chattering had been so agonizing, and now it was gone. But so was another piece of Jon.

Maggie was again grieved at the waste, permitting the flow of tears once more. As the wave lulled, she gratefully drew up her resolve again, returning to the prophesying chart. The next mile marker of stage 7 read "nonambulatory." Jon still walked, but his knees would not straighten completely, and she often had to prompt him to shift his weight and take another step. She walked behind him always, praying that he would not fall on her.

She scanned the remaining symptoms and saw an uneasy picture of Jon's disease forming in front of her. To her dismay, there was also a companion image, a memory pushing its way up, a very old thing that had no place here and which she had no desire to revisit. Thankfully, she heard Jon on the move and was able to push the thing aside. It was definitely best to not think about that one right now.

She hurried down the hall to help Jon, who had walked himself to the bathroom. Thank goodness, he had kept the pull-up on all night! But she had a dilly of a time getting the drawstring untied, Jon leaning on her as she balanced him precariously with one shoulder while her hands struggled with the knot. "Where are we going, Jon?" she murmured from under his heavy form.

"Is my dad coming over today?" was the response.

And Maggie worked to keep Jon up and her fears down.

Maggie's Nightmare

The days rushed, and the nights dragged, and the insistent old memory visited Maggie more and more. One sleepless night, she could block the image no longer. A memory of her mother crowded its way past her weakened defenses. A distorted face, familiar gray hair tangled and spilling over a stretcher pillow, eyes sedated but still wild, about to be lifted into the ambulance for transfer to a nursing home, her mental illness and lifestyle choices finally catching up with her.

"Don't let them put me in the nursing home, Maggie," the slurred voice begged. "They kill old people with their morphine." Because of her mother's mental illness, Maggie had grown up around dozens of paranoid ideations. She had no idea why this particular one was shoving its way forward. Well, perhaps she did.

> *Old messages and their influences*

She tried again to push the picture of her mother and the nursing home away from her, but some things just cannot be unseen. She supposed time would have to tell.

And time responded loudly a few weeks later, as Maggie was walking with Jon to the bedroom. He quite unexpectedly sat himself down in the middle of the hallway and would not budge. Maggie begged and pushed and pulled, but Jon was done for the day. She finally surrendered and brought him blankets and a pillow. Jon slept all night on the floor, and Maggie was forced to call the neighbor the next morning to drag and lift Jon into the bed. She sat beside him for a while and for the first time brought legitimacy to the fear that she had made her husband a promise that she might not be able to keep.

The Crossroads

Maggie called the doctor's office that same morning, and their old friend came right to the phone. He was kind and sympathetic, having cared for the couple for many years and being familiar with their peculiarities. He listened to Maggie describe Jon's changes, but he had little to offer in the way of treatments, as she expected by now. He asked her the next obvious question—was Jon safe to be at home? Maggie wavered and then hedged, "What if he isn't? What can we do?" The doctor offered her his best advice: nursing home placement.

And just like that, her mother's words popped out of her own mouth. "I don't want the nurses there to kill him with their medicines," the voice in her head announced out loud.

"Ahh," she heard her friend chuckle, a tease in his voice. "The old morphine rumor. I sure wish I knew where that one got started. But I promise that I won't let anyone kill your husband, Maggie. Does that make you feel better?" She could imagine his wrinkled old face grinning as he said it, and she was more than a little embarrassed. But she pushed on, wanting to be clear.

> Morphine: truths and rumors

"Oh, I suppose so. But nonetheless, I don't want them to give him any medicines that might hurry it along."

"Agreed," the doctor fielded. "And just to reassure you, Maggie, if I do order any pain medicine for Jon, it works in the same general way as the painkillers I ordered for you when you broke your wrist, remember? It's a little early for this conversation, Maggie, but we're old friends, and I do want you to be aware of what might be down the road. Dying can be hard for some, dear. Understand that the medicines can help at the end, but they don't cause the end. The end is there anyway. Does that make some sense?" He stopped, waiting for Maggie to speak, but she didn't.

"Tell you what. Let me call a hospice agency to talk to you. Maybe they can help you make some decisions about what to do with Jon. And in the meantime, go visit a few nursing homes. There comes a time, Maggie, when we have moved through all of our best choices, and we just have to be glad that there is another choice available to us."

Maggie mumbled something noncommittal and hung up the phone, the wind blown out of her sails. It was coming to this: hospice, nursing homes, and death. She sighed as she heard Jon turn in bed. They were both so tired. Maggie walked toward the bedroom, just wanting their old life back.

Caregiver Syndrome

A hospice nurse rang the doorbell the next morning, and Maggie showed her in. Between Jon's mumbling in one ear and her mother's warnings in the other, Maggie had not slept again. She made a cup of coffee for herself and one for the nurse and tried to answer the questions as best she could.

Was there more family? No.

Would she want to employ a sitter to come into their home? Absolutely not.

Could she afford a nursing home for Jon? Maybe, there was a life insurance policy.

Would she like help with placement?

At that, Maggie fell apart, unexpectedly and without her permission. This was so unlike her, she explained to the nurse through her tears. But her resolve had become more like Swiss cheese these days, with more holes than solid surface. The nurse allowed her the moment and then described "caregiver syndrome" to her, and Maggie conceded that she was experiencing nearly every symptom. The nurse offered a temporary solution, suggesting that Maggie take advantage of hospice respite care. She explained that in certain circumstances, hospice would place a patient in a nursing home for a few days for the purpose of giving the caregiver a chance to rest and recover. Maggie dug her fingers into her palms. Then releasing them, she reluctantly agreed to the nurse's suggestion. She was weary to the bone and found herself trying on the unfamiliar idea of being grateful that there was another choice available to her, as her friend had suggested.

> Caregiver syndrome and Respite

Jon Goes to Respite

It was an emotional morning when the ambulance came to pick up Jon. Maggie couldn't remember a time when they'd slept apart. This was temporary, she told herself, as she followed the ambulance in her car. Breckenwood Manor was painted on the sign above the door, the paint peeling and a smell of disinfectant hitting her senses as she walked into the lobby. Residents wheeled themselves along the corridor walls, a haphazard parade of lost stares and mismatched clothes. They looked clean but not kempt, she weighed. Some of the nurses looked harried; others appeared bored. The manor looked tired and running on low fuel—much like she herself felt.

Jon was placed in the bed nearest the window. It was not a private room, but the roommate was absent, his side of the room surprisingly decorated and welcoming. Jon did not look concerned after his ride in the ambulance. He just lay in his new bed looking at the ceiling. He was agitated when he became aware of Maggie, however, asking for his father, asking when supper was. She held his hand and answered his questions again and again, until he was finally reassured enough to lean back against the pillows, his eyes returning to the ceiling. Maggie finished the admission process with the intake nurse and stepped out quietly as Jon was being fed his supper by an attendant. All she had left was to hope that they would take good care of him.

Maggie drove home and walked into the empty house. She stayed busy scheduling doctors' appointments for herself and a much-needed salon day and then fell into bed dreaming of a full night's sleep. But the morning found her groggy; her mind overburdened and unable to shut off, wondering how Jon had fared overnight. She scrambled some eggs as she called the nursing home to check on him. Her phone call was rerouted several times before the correct nursing station picked it up. Apparently, Jon had not slept well either and had required a sleeping pill and later antianxiety medication. He had finally fallen asleep about 3:00 a.m., per the night shift report. But he was wide awake now and was being fed his breakfast. She thanked the nurse and hung up. Well, Maggie thought, it would have to do.

Nursing Home Decision

The days passed more quickly than Maggie imagined they could, and soon, it was decision time. Maggie had seen her cardiologist, had her hair done, and had visited the two remaining nursing homes in town. When the hospice social worker called a few days later, Maggie's decision had been made—not because it was her favorite choice, but because the choices were so few. One nursing home was nicer but was too far away for her to drive. The other was too expensive, and she would be using much of their savings as it was. She'd contemplated keeping Jon at home with hospice help, but she was just not strong enough to care for a bedridden Jon. No, she would have to ask Jon's forgiveness for not keeping her promise, and she would do the next best thing, which would be to visit him every day.

> *When staying home is no longer possible*

"One of the values that you can regain," the social worker had shared, sensitive to Maggie's dilemma, "is that you can return to being his wife again, rather than caregiver, bath aide, cook, janitor, safety coordinator, and every other duty that has taken you away from the one role that only you *can* provide him. You will still be able to love him, Maggie, just in a different way." Yes, Maggie supposed, it would have to do.

A Journey of One

Jon did not return home but stayed on, now as a resident of Breckenwood Manor. Maggie arrived every morning to feed him breakfast and then returned again to feed him supper and watch TV with him until he fell asleep. During the day, Jon attended some of the scheduled activities, sitting and rocking in his wheelchair. He never participated, but he did seem to enjoy the bustle and the snacks. His roommate discovered that Jon perked up when he played swing band tunes on his old CD player, and he would turn up the volume for Jon, enjoying the smile on his face and the off-beat tap of Jon's hand on the bedrail.

Weeks passed, and Maggie eventually slept through the night. She had received a thorough chastising from her cardiologist for her swollen ankles, but in the end, a few medication adjustments were made, and her symptoms improved. She had developed a comfortable pattern at the nursing home, and Jon was doing well—or at least well enough. So she was surprised when the hospice nurse called her early one afternoon.

Jon Slips Away Home

"Mrs. MacDouglas?" The nurse's voice was hesitant. And she had not used her last name since Maggie had nipped that at their initial visit. "The nursing home called me about an hour ago. I'm here now. Can you take a seat somewhere while I talk to you?"

Maggie's nerves hissed. Was this going to be "the" phone call? She had seen Jon just a few hours ago, and he had been fine.

"What's wrong?" she asked, sharper than she meant to. She heard a long exhale on the other end.

"He has slipped away, Maggie. It couldn't have been any easier on him. He was listening to his neighbor's music, and when the attendant came in next, he had simply passed. I'm so sorry, Maggie. This is such hard news to tell you. I'm surprised myself—I thought he'd be with us a little longer." She paused for Maggie's response, but Maggie didn't seem to have one. She was numb.

"Maggie? Are you all right?" the nurse asked, concern in her voice.

"Yes, I'm here. I'm just having a hard time believing this. I saw him this morning, and he was fine." Then, she said, "I'm on my way." And she hung the phone up abruptly.

Bewildered, Maggie grabbed her keys. She would have had some sort of premonition, or warning, wouldn't she? Had she even kissed him when she left this morning? She couldn't remember.

He wasn't dead; he just couldn't be. She made herself slow down. She couldn't abide a dizzy spell right now. She had to go see Jon. He would be sitting up in bed as usual. And this time, he might even smile at her.

That was the thought she held as she backed down the driveway, cutting the gravel edge a little close. And she would give them all a piece of her mind too for scaring her so. Once on the straight road, however, her mind wondered. *He's been on hospice, Maggie, and that means he was near his end. That was the hospice nurse on the phone, Maggie. She knows death when she sees it.* But it was so hard to imagine. She'd seen him alive a million times, but she'd never seen him dead. She wouldn't think about it, she told herself, as the Manor came into view.

She weaved into the parking lot to see the hospice nurse scurrying toward her, an empty wheelchair in tow. She looked more than harried.

"Maggie," she scolded, "I didn't want you to drive yourself—here, I brought this for you. We've got your heart to think about too. Let me wheel you to him." And she effectively scooped Maggie's small body into the wheelchair before she could utter a protest. She reached over and pulled the keys out of the ignition, handing them to Maggie with one hand as she whirled the chair around with the other, navigating them off the parking lot. The antiseptic smell hit Maggie, as it always did. She anticipated flying down the hallway at a breakneck speed, but instead, the nurse detoured the wheelchair into the waiting area. Maggie found herself knee to knee with a waiting room chair as the nurse slid herself into it, grabbing Maggie's hands. Her hands were cool, and she didn't speak for a moment, collecting herself. The lobby was empty, and the receptionist took her cue, sliding closed the glass window.

> Death comes early sometimes

"Maggie," the nurse looked kindly but pointedly into Maggie's face. "He really is gone—I've seen him. We'll go back there in a moment, but I want you to hear me, that he really has passed. As hard as it is at this time, maybe later we'll be able to see the blessing in it, that he didn't have to suffer all the way to the end. Today was his day to go home, Maggie. There was nothing else that could be done. You did well by him. He knew that you loved him, and that was what mattered. You gave him your most valued treasures—your time and your heart. He felt loved and cared for, Maggie. You showed him that very well." The nurse stopped her reassurances, searching Maggie's eyes for acceptance of the truths that she had laid out.

A lovely poison, Maggie thought. "*Your husband is dead, but he was loved.*"

She felt her heart clench closed. These were nice sentiments, but if Jon was dead, then her heart was dead also. She had dedicated everything to him, and he was the only world she had. If she loosed her heart right now, her insides would melt out like butter. *No, better to keep a tight check on things and not think too hard. Better to just keep moving.*

Maggie's Denial

"I want to see him," Maggie snapped, her lips a thin line, her eyes leveled at the door to the hallway.

"All right," the nurse relented, rising. "I'll take you there. They've moved his roommate to another room so that we can have some privacy. But we're going to go there slowly. I'm more than a little worried about you." She turned the wheelchair and worked it calmly but deliberately through the passageways. Maggie noticed no change in the regular residents. They still paddled their wheelchairs aimlessly on their way to who knew where. But the staff seemed different. There were sad smiles on a few, and others seemed to find something important to do as she was wheeled by. They finally made the turn to her husband's hallway, and Maggie realized that her heart was racing. She gulped in a breath, sensing an uneasy hollowness in her soul, painful to its depth. Her insides

> Denial
> Anger
> Bargaining
> Depression
> and back
> again

began their melt against all of her will, wrenching up into her throat, which tightened and held. She drew wheezes of air sharply in through her nose, hot and stinging. Surrendering, her chest released a shattering sob, and her hands fluttered at the nurse to stop. Maggie had been so determined to step into that room and see her husband sitting up, smiling, and holding his hand out to her. But now she was afraid to go near, afraid to look at his face, to see it frozen forever in its death mask.

She gasped out a few more sobs—quick, heaving ones. Surprising ones. Somehow, as they had made the last turn, she had known for herself that Jon was indeed gone. Beyond that closed door up ahead, Jon was truly dead.

The wave of pain took its time, but it finally released enough for Maggie to motion her hand weakly to resume the procession. Maggie observed that the hospice chaplain had arrived and was following reverently behind them, her black skirt swishing. That made it official.

Jon's Not Here

The nurse pushed open the room door, and Maggie found herself in the familiar room. The nurse reached across to lock the wheels of the chair and then held her hand out to Maggie, whose gaze had narrowed to the tiles at her feet. Tan and white, white and tan.

"We're here."

The nurse touched her hand and gently helped her up, steadying her. She was guided over to the chair that had been placed at the head of Jon's bed. She counted the tiles on her way and then cautiously lowered herself to the chair edge. Her eyes moved warily from the floor up to the bedrail and then to the edge of the coverlet. They lingered on the pattern for a moment and then finally lifted to the pale face that lay still against the pillow. Jon? The form was definitely dead, no doubt about that. But it didn't look like Jon. Well, she supposed it did in a fashion. Those were his long fingers stretched out on his chest, but there was no spark on the face at all. And oddly not a familiar wrinkle either; he was as smooth as baby skin. She studied the face closer. This body, this form—this unplugged mannequin—was not Jon. Her Jon was obviously not in there anymore. Remarkable, how empty it looked. Where was her husband? And why didn't this part hurt? She'd been stabbed as if by a knife just outside the room. But this was, well, there was only one word for it—finished. There was no Jon here to mourn or to worry about. Then the stab did hit again, sharp and deep. There was no one to love her or worry about her either. Tears came freely now, causing the nurse and chaplain to move closer, not wanting to interfere with her grief but to comfort if they could.

As the tears loosened the last of her restraints, Maggie finally released the reins.

"I thought I was prepared!" she lashed out. "I can't believe that it's all over. It was so much, and now he's gone! We had so much time together, but it isn't enough. I want more. I don't want him to be gone." She stood up and turned away, stumbling, but the chaplain was there to grasp her arm. She was seasoned and had been watching for the cathartic signs of breakthrough, as painful as they were to experience and to watch.

"I can't take this! I just can't take it," Maggie cried into the chaplain's shoulder. A handkerchief was discreetly pressed into her hand.

The chaplain held her quietly. "I've arranged a private room for us down the hall, if you'd like to go sit there, Maggie. We'll take as much time as you need, and when you're ready, we'll ask the nurse to call the funeral home …"

"Oh, you can call them now," Maggie lifted her head. "He's not in there. He's not in there at all. That's just the shell. It's so odd, how true that is right now. It's all I've got left of him, but it's not really him. Go ahead and call the funeral home. I just want to go home. You go ahead and call who you need to. I'm leaving." And with that, Maggie was out the door, the chaplain surprised and rushing quickly to catch up with her. It had been prearranged that the chaplain would escort Maggie back to her home while the nurse waited for the funeral home transport team to arrive. But Maggie was calling the shots, and they did their best to keep up.

The chaplain was grudgingly allowed into the house when Maggie saw that she had been tailed. Maggie was all business again, though her eyes showed an emptiness that staying busy could not disguise. She called her daughter-in-law and informed her of Jon's death. There was no other family to notify. Jon was to have a small graveside service, and Maggie asked the chaplain if she would preside. She then notified the neighbors of her husband's passing, and the next day, two casseroles arrived with condolence cards.

Maggie's Story

Maggie lived alone at home for the next five years, eventually paying one of the neighbors to clean and grocery shop for her. One Fall morning, she called Breckenwood Manor and asked how to get herself admitted, stating that she could no longer manage by herself at home. Maggie called her daughter-in-law to inform her of her plans, relaying that the house, which she would inherit at Maggie's death, was soon to be vacant and that she could do with it as she willed, including all the items inside. She hated to leave her daughter-in-law with such a task, but, well, it was better if they just didn't talk about that. Maggie lived the remainder of her life at Breckenwood Manor, passing away the following year under the care of the same hospice agency. In a small graveside service, as the leaves were beginning their change, Maggie was laid to rest next to her beloved Jon.

> Acceptance: going it alone

Jonas MacDouglas, aged eighty-eight, passed away peacefully at Breckenwood Manor nursing home, hospice bereavement services to follow.

Magdelene MacDouglas, aged eighty-three, also of Breckenwood Manor, joined her husband in death following a six-year bereavement.

QUESTIONS FOR REFLECTION
CHAPTER 3: JON

1. One in ten people age sixty-five and older has Alzheimer's dementia. Who in your family has dementia, and how does it affect the family?

2. Doctors and medical personnel always teach us to keep our loved one oriented and in touch with reality so as to promote mental health. But at some point, Maggie realizes that Jon's mental losses have overcome his ability to understand his environment and that her constant correcting is more stressful than beneficial for both. Does it feel to you that Maggie gave up? How do you think their son, had he lived, would have felt if he came home to find empty drawers, deadbolts on doors, a urine smell in the corners, and his mother agreeing with his father's delusions, rather than continuing her attempts to stop the disease progression?

3. Caregiver syndrome is real, but it can be prevented, or at least lightened. Family calendars, a willingness to ask for help, permission to take breaks, lower expectations, and so on can make a difference. Are you or someone you know suffering from caregiver syndrome? What steps can be taken to lighten your load? It has been suggested that it takes six people to care for one ill person to prevent caregiver burnout. Do you have six people in your life who will come to your support should you need them? If not, what steps can you take now to develop these relationships?

4. Jon's illness triggered old memories of Maggie's mother and her illness. Does it surprise you that, in times of stress, old messages that have been deeply buried can resurface and complicate a current situation?

5. Maggie's mother believed that nursing homes and hospices use morphine to hasten death. While it is true that medications can relax a body, making it easier to let go, pain and anxiety are stressors that also tend to shorten life. But did you know that people who receive hospice care live an average of twenty-nine days longer than those who do not?[1] How do you feel about having comfort medications when it is your time to die? What about when it is your loved one's time to die?

---

[1] 1 Stephen R. Connor, PhD, Bruce Pyenson, FSA, MAAA, Kathryn Fitch, RN, MA, MEd, Carol Spence, RN, MS, and Kosuke Iwasaki, FIAJ, MAAA, "Comparing Hospice and Nonhospice Patient Survival among Patients Who Die within a Three-Year Window," Journal of Pain and Symptom Management 33 no. (3 March 2007): 238.

CHAPTER 4

Martina's Journey

- Age 46, cancer
- Primary symptom: terminal agitation
- Primary caregivers: Nina (26) and Julian (24)

The Road Together

Martina and Her Family

Martina Rose is a forty-six-year-old divorced female with lung cancer in its last stages. Martina was diagnosed one year ago and elected for chemotherapy and radiation with a brief remission achieved. But the cancer is back with a vengeance and has spread. Martina recently moved in with her daughter, Nina, a stay-at-home mom of two preschool girls. Nina's husband is a mechanic at a nearby garage and has been able to adjust his hours to provide more help at home. Martina also has a son, Julian, who is single and two years younger than Nina. He makes the trip across town several evenings a week to visit his mother and to get a home-cooked meal at Nina's house. This system worked well while Martina was self-sufficient, but Martina's condition is changing. She tires easily now and is often short of breath. Nina watches and worries as her mother holds on to furniture and chairs, sitting down often to catch her breath. But something even more unsettling is happening to Martina.

The Path Bends

Julian, who hasn't seen his mother in several days, has remarked that her color has changed, though the rest of the family does not see it. Nina notes some new confusion in the morning, coming in to find her mother tugging at her nightgown, seemingly having forgotten how to manage the buttons. She also tosses and turns at night, twisting blankets and sheets into knots as she drifts in and out of shallow sleep. But she sleeps just fine during the day, which annoys Nina, though she wants to feel more gracious about it. Her mother's short catnap has become something more akin to a mini-coma. She wonders if the daytime activity and background noise of the children helps her mother feel more secure to sleep. But Nina needs her sleep too, and she's having trouble attending to her mother's wakefulness at night and then being a full-on mom during the day. Regardless of the reason, Nina's energy has run thin, and she doesn't know if she can keep up this pace.

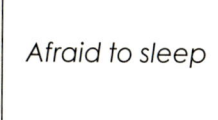

> Afraid to sleep

Martina has been especially peculiar in the past few days. She has always been headstrong and determined, but lately, she has been downright irritable! She is uncharacteristically cranky with the girls and even swatted at Nina when she tried to help with the nightgown. Nothing is the same about her. She has stopped eating breakfast and only nibbles at lunch and dinner, and she won't wear her oxygen at all. And the arguments over the most obvious things! It is not morning yet, there is water already at your bedside, the girls are not crying … Was Nina losing her mind, or was her mother?

No One Is Sleeping

The following two weeks felt as if the family was on a nonstop merry-go-round that had no off switch. Nina was functioning in a thick fog herself now, trying to keep up with her children by day and her mother by night. The two men helped as they were able, but they were limited by their jobs. Everyone was on twenty-four-hour patrol. Except for her long afternoon naps, Martina seemed unable to sleep at all now. She looked so very tired and fragile. She went straight to bed at night but was up again within the hour. Nina would look up to find her standing in the doorway, legs wobbling impossibly. She could only jump up and run, praying that she would reach her mother before she fell. But Nina wasn't always fast enough, and bruises and skin tears soon decorated Martina's wasting legs and forearms, the skin beneath the bruises eerily opaque. Nina saw but could not believe that this was her strong, lively mother, who had been working full-time just three months ago. She looked more like pictures of her grandmother or even her great-grandmother. She could count Martina's ribs and noticed now how the muscles between them pulled with each breath.

> Terminal agitation

The House Is Quiet

One morning, Nina woke to a too-quiet house. Had her mother finally slept through the night? Or was it something else? Maybe she had fallen, or maybe she was in the bed and ...

Nina sat up quickly, listening; knowing that she should rush to her mother's room but unable to make herself move, afraid of what she might find. She picked up the phone to ask her husband to come home but set it back down again. No, she should be able to do this herself. She had seen her mother act with courage through this disease, and she should try to do the same. She eased into her robe, calling her mother's name softly as she walked down the hallway, afraid of waking the girls in the adjoining room. She heard no answer. As she approached the doorway, she exhaled in relief, hearing a soft snore coming from her

> Caregiver fears

mother's bed. Walking hurriedly now, she reached out for her mother's hand. It was not cold as she had feared but was wonderfully warm, if a little moist. She looked to see that her mother's chest was rising and falling, a recently acquired habit. Nina was thankful. Martina was finally getting a good night's sleep. Her mouth was open (unusually wide, Nina thought), and there was a low rattle in her throat. She bent her head closer, listening to the wet congestion, and wondered if her mother had somehow contracted pneumonia.

Nina shook her mother's arm gently. Martina did not open her eyes. She shook harder, calling her name now, but there was no response. In a panic, Nina pinched her on the arm like she might do to get a child's attention, but there was not even a flinch of Martina's eyelids. She ran back to her bedroom for the phone and this time did call her husband. Then she called Julian. Their mutual advice was to call the doctor, quickly.

The Crossroads

Hard Decisions: How Best to Love

As the receptionist at the oncologist's office answered, Nina's words rushed to tell her of her mother's unresponsiveness. The receptionist picked up on the urgency and asked if Nina wanted an ambulance. Her first response was to accept any and all help, but then she hesitated. The last time they were at the hospital, her mother had begged them not to bring her there again. But they had not talked about it further.

> Home or hospital

"Will the ambulance take her back to the hospital?" Nina had no idea what was the right thing to do. She just knew that her mother wasn't waking up, and that had her scared.

"Usually, yes," the receptionist answered cautiously, hearing the tremble in Nina's voice. "Isn't that what you want?"

Nina tried to call up the courage that she had found earlier. "No," she answered finally. "Mom said she didn't want to go back to the hospital. Could you send a nurse or someone out?"

The receptionist asked her to hold while she paged the office nurse to the phone.

"Nina, is this you? Martina's daughter?" A familiar voice was on the line. The nurse's southern intonation was thick, recalling her to memory from Martina's many office visits. Nina confirmed and launched into her story again.

"I'm so sorry, Nina, but we don't do home visits from this office. We will be glad to refer you to a hospice agency if you'd like. They are usually able to send a nurse out the same day."

Nina remembered a previous offer of hospice, but her mother had dismissed it outright. Despite what the doctors were telling them, dying had been an unthinkable outcome at that time. She found herself temporarily lost in the memories and traumas of the last year, and she worked to pull herself back to the present.

"I think it might be a good idea now. Will they come to the house?"

"Yes, hon, they go wherever the patient is." The musical accent soothed somehow. "I'll make a few phone calls and will get right back to you. Are you okay being there, honey? Is anyone there with you?" This nurse loved endearments.

"My husband is on his way home," Nina assured her, straightening. Her ears had picked up another sing-song voice, this one coming from the children's bedroom. Her time was about to be divided again. "I'm fine, I guess. Mom's just lying there, so there's nothing that we can do for her right now. It's just so different from what she's been like lately."

Then a terrible thought arose.

"What if Mom stops breathing? What do I do?" Nina gushed, afraid again. The nurse didn't answer, but Nina could hear the click of fingernails on computer keys. When she spoke again, her voice was uneasy, as if about to give more bad news.

"Her chart states that she wants a full code, Nina, which means that she wants everything done to try to bring her back to life." She paused then, breathing quietly. A nail tip was heard tapping the desk. She seemed to be contemplating how much to say.

"I'm going to tell you something personal, Nina, based on all of my experiences." Her tone softened. "I'm going to encourage you to rethink this, especially now that things seem to have changed. Television has made us believe that everybody lives after CPR, but the facts are more like 6 percent when it's a home resuscitation. It's less than 20 percent even if CPR is started right there in the hospital.[2] Now this is only my opinion, but I've seen a lot of things in my job, working with families who are right where you are. This decision was made at a different time of life. The choice to change her from CPR to DNR seems hard at this moment, but if left as it stands now, the results of the decision may be even harder."

Nina was listening, but both girls were awake now, their small voices singing and talking to their dolls, their fingers, the ceiling. She couldn't believe she was having this dark conversation with sweet cherub sounds in the background. There was something poignant here, but she was too unnerved to catch it.

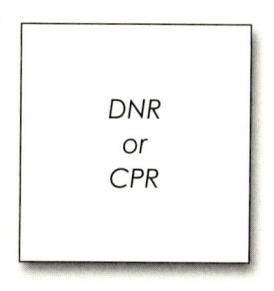

> DNR or CPR

"What do you mean?" Nina asked, glancing toward the bedrooms.

"Do you want me to be honest, or will this be too much for you?" The nurse was truly asking.

Nina took a deep breath and told the nurse to be honest. She guessed it was finally time to know what they were dealing with. But her mind was whirling. Was Mom dying, or was she not? Should they resuscitate, or should they not? Would the girls be impacted horribly if they saw their grandmother resuscitated, or would dying in her room be any better? Nina had no experience with this. What had they all been thinking?

---

[2] "Key CPR Facts and Stats 2018–2019" (2019, February), retrieved from http://cprcertificationonlinehq.com/cpr-facts-stats/.

The nurse took her cue, speaking clearly, steadily.

"In my thirty years of experience as a nurse, I've come to the conclusion that just because we *can* do CPR doesn't always mean that we should. If a person has a healthy body to come back to, well, that is certainly one thing. But your mother would only come back to another day of cancer and now with tubes and a ventilator and quite possibly broken ribs and internal organ damage. Families don't often know the medical side of it—they're just doing their best to make decisions out of love. But sometimes letting a body take its natural course is another way to love. Of course, this is a decision that *your* family has to make, and I won't do anything to talk you out of it. I just want you to have all the facts so that you can make an educated decision that you can live with. You are her advocate now and need to do what you think is best for her."

She stopped and then decided to go forward and speak her last sentence.

"If the 6 percent even worked, Nina, it would only bring her back to have to die again." The nurse was silent then, letting Nina and the weighty message rest for a moment. Hard news on top of bad news.

Nina stood, listening, deciding—her body shaking.

"Can we change our minds back again later?" Her voice was small, no stronger than the toddlers' down the hall. The nurse's last sentence had numbed her brain.

On the other end of the phone, the nurse narrowed her attention from the chaos of the doctor's office behind her to only Nina at the other end of the line. She had seen so many family tragedies in her years of oncology.

"It feels like betrayal to let her go, doesn't it, angel?" she offered gently. "But as an old nurse, I can assure you that it's only betrayal if your motives are greater for yourself than they are for your mother. And I just don't hear that in you, Nina. Death is the natural outcome of life, honey. I'm so sorry that this is happening to you. You are being asked to make decisions that many gray-headed folks have never had to make. I'm just wanting to start this conversation with you, so that your family can be thinking about it while you wait for the hospice nurse. I'm sure she'll talk with you more about it when she arrives."

The noises from the girls' room had escalated from quiet singing to urgent requests to be picked up and get their day started, but the nurse had more to say. Her words remained measured, but she had switched now to her teaching voice.

"Your mother's cancer is definitely terminal, dear. The doctor told her so at the last visit, but I wasn't sure that she was hearing him. I'll tell the hospice nurse to hurry on out. Until then, don't try to give your mother anything to eat or drink unless she's fully awake and sitting up. Raise the head of her bed and put her oxygen on if she's having any trouble breathing. She can probably still hear you, so talk to her and tell her that you love her and that she is doing great. And tell her that you guys are also doing fine, if you think it's true enough to tell her. That's the best message a mother can hear from her children."

Nina's voice strangled, not sure of that last part. "I'll try," was all she could manage.

"You're doing a great job, love. Hang in there. And I'm sorry, but I've got one last difficult question to ask you. Has your mother made any funeral arrangements?"

Funeral arrangements? No, they had never talked about funeral arrangements. They had barely talked about the cancer. Nina only knew that her mother's bank account was empty and that there was no money saved for a funeral.

"No, we didn't think she was that close. Will hospice pay for the funeral?"

"No, darling, I'm afraid not; funerals are paid by the families. But hospice can help you

> Hospice and funerals

decide your options. You start talking things over with your family while I make my phone calls. I'll call you back when I know their arrival time."

Nina thanked her and hung up, grateful to be done with the

phone call and even more grateful to see her husband walk through the front door. The girls heard him as well and called out, but he came to Nina first, arms open to encircle her. Nina leaned in, savoring the momentary comfort as she spilled out the conversation she'd just had. Her stoicism unraveled like a loose thread opening a seam.

"They're going to send out a hospice nurse, and there are no funeral arrangements; Mom won't wake up, and the girls want up, and I don't want to think about my mother dying, and …" Her words left her and shudders and sobs took their place. She was still upright by simple will alone.

"I'll get the girls dressed and take them out," her husband consoled, patting her back and kissing her wet cheek, his rough hand brushing down her lumpy, uncombed hair. She smelled the gasoline and grease of his uniform and felt grounded by the familiarity.

"You go sit with your mother and wait for the nurse. We'll get through this, Nin'. We always do." He kissed her forehead and then released her, calling out to the girls that he was on his way. He peered into Martina's room as he passed by and gave Nina a reassuring signal that she was still with them.

Unprepared

Nina washed her face and brushed her hair and then walked back to her mother's room, her mind pondering the information from the doctor's office. She recalled that last appointment at the doctor's office. Her mother had been coughing up blood, but that had not been unusual. She had still been working and had even driven them to the appointment. But she had insisted that Nina stay in the waiting room while she saw the doctor. On the way home, her mother would only say that the cancer was back and that it had spread. That was all she would say. Nina remembered questioning her about more chemotherapy or radiation, but her mother had simply said that it would not help and that had been that. There was no sense in asking about it further; this was her mother's way. And, Nina now realized, she herself had been a willing accomplice with the silence and wishful thinking.

She supposed that her mother had not wanted to upset her and Julian. But if she had been told she was going to die, wouldn't it have been better for them to have talked about it? Shouldn't they have been a little more prepared? Now Mom was comatose in bed, and what if she never woke up again? They had not even said goodbye!

Nina pulled a chair up to the bed, watching her mother's face. There was no change. Her mother still snored lightly, the rattle low in her throat. Her yellowed hand rose and fell on her chest. Nina sat and watched—and waited for hospice.

Hospice and the Talk

When the nurse arrived, Julian was right behind her, actually beside her and pushing past her in his hurry to get to his mother's room. Nina spilled out her story again, recounting the last horrible weeks—her mother's restlessness, how she picked at her clothes and at her bedcovers, even grasping at invisible objects in the air. She detailed all the confused conversations and how Mom had argued and hit at them. The nurse listened, nodding her head with understanding as Nina unloaded.

"You might be describing a common end-of-life symptom," the nurse began when Nina was finished.

There it was again, another medical term that screamed, "Brace yourself, Nina."

"We call it terminal restlessness," the nurse continued as she guided Nina to the couch. She quietly moved toys and laundry over to make a space.

"It happens for several reasons, but the basics are that oxygen levels are falling and metabolic toxins are being released as the body systems slow down."

Nina wanted to shut her ears, but the nurse prattled on,

reassuring her that she would first look for other causes of her mother's restlessness, such as pain, constipation, bladder retention, or infection. She informed her that there were sedatives that could be given to help relieve her mother's mind and keep her safe. And she warned that they should not leave her alone, in case she woke up and tried to get out of bed. Nina tuned back in to the conversation.

"She's not that way anymore. It's like she's in a coma or something." Nina re-explained, wondering if the nurse had missed that part.

"I've seen patients who have been in bed for months, then suddenly they are in the kitchen trying to prepare dinner."

Nina was shocked by this but vaguely encouraged that her mother might wake up again. By this time, Julian was stepping out of the bedroom and heading toward them.

"I've seen the reports that the doctor's office sent over, and you've given me a good description of what she's been like lately," the nurse said, standing and giving Julian her seat. "So let me go see Mrs. Rose now, and then we'll talk again. You're welcome to come join me, or you can remain here."

The siblings opted for the couch.

The nurse crossed the room to their mother's doorway and then knocked and courteously asked if she could enter. They heard her moving about the room, turning on a lamp, speaking politely to their unresponsive mother, telling her what she was about to do, encouraging her as she took her blood pressure, and apologizing as she turned her, reassuring her that she was keeping her backside well-covered and saying that she hoped she was not causing any pain. After several minutes, they heard the lamp click off, and soon, the nurse was walking back to them, her face neutral and unreadable. She pulled over a chair from the kitchen and sat to face the young-adult children of Mrs. Rose. The two sat close to each other, their hands folded in their laps, dread and

"The talk"

expectancy in battle on each face. The nurse took a breath in for herself and began "the talk."

"I can tell that your mother has been fighting very hard," she initiated, "and I can see that this sudden change is a surprise for you. Cancer can be deceiving. It doesn't look too bad at first, and people are usually able to carry on their lives almost normally. They are more tired and don't feel their best, but they keep functioning and are able to push on with only a little compromise. But the cancer cells are always working in their body, stealing energy and nutrients. Eventually, there is little left for the body to use for itself." She paused a brief moment. "That is what I'm seeing in your mother. There's just not much left to fight with." Nina's face had stonewalled, shutting off, but Julian was leaning forward and listening intently.

"Sis told me that she's warm and that there is a rattling in her chest. Should she be on antibiotics?" His eyes were hopeful or perhaps desperate.

"The rattling that we hear in her chest isn't from infection." The nurse was careful, choosing her words. "This is a normal process that happens near the end of life. She has a bit of a fever as well, but that's not from infection either. It's from dehydration and from the toxins that I mentioned earlier."

> Identifying end-of-life symptoms

"So you'll put her on IVs," Julian broke in, understanding that this was the usual treatment for dehydration.

The nurse pressed her lips together, wondering how much these two young people would be able to grasp in just this first visit. But she also wasn't sure how many more visits there would be for Mrs. Rose. She chose not to hold back, even if her message was hard for them to hear. She didn't want this family to have unfounded regrets later that their mother might have lived "if only we had ..." She simplified the next explanations as best she could, weighing what they did not know against how much they could take in.

"I wish that would work, Julian, but it would only make things worse in the long run. Your mother's brain has shut down her desire to eat or drink. Her body can't handle anything more important than keeping her heart and lungs going. The processing of food and water takes a lot of energy, and her body knows what it needs to do. IV fluids might perk her up for a day or two, but then what would happen to all that fluid? The fluid would go everywhere that it's not supposed to be—mostly into the lungs, which can make breathing very difficult. That's why we don't hydrate at the end of life. It may correct one problem for the moment, but it creates a landslide of others."

She paused, waiting to see that Julian was still with her. He was, so she pressed on.

"Let me share something else with you, and this may sound obvious, but I want you to remember that what your body needs and what your mother's body needs right now are very different. Can you keep an open mind about that for a moment?"

Julian nodded that he was trying.

"We don't think of it this way for our bodies, but in your mother's body, dehydration isn't all bad. It creates a haziness of the mind and causes sleepiness and malaise. These are natural events that can help the passing to be a little easier." The nurse looked at Julian to see if he accepted this. She hoped Nina was listening as well, but she showed no signs, staring absently into her hands. Julian, however, was fully engaged now and was obviously not liking what he was hearing. He edged forward in his seat, jumping several steps ahead in the conversation.

"But shouldn't we try to keep her awake? If she sleeps, won't she die sooner?" His lower lip betrayed a miniscule quiver, but he kept his eyes locked to hers. Tears collected unwillingly at their corners, and he blinked them back, once, twice.

Julian was grasping the more important message. But seeing the struggle of the boy made it hard for even a toughened hospice nurse to keep her tears at bay. Her eyes moistened as she worked to maintain composure, respecting Julian and his brave restraint.

"I can see how much you want to keep her with you, Julian. And for you, every second with her counts. But for her, it's different. She's very tired. I'm convinced that she loves you children more than life itself; I can tell by the love and dedication that you are giving back to her. But your mother is experiencing this through different eyes."

Keeping Them Here; Letting Them Go

"There's a turn that the dying must make, like the turn of a road. They know they can't stay here, and the effort to work at it is eventually too much; the relief of rest becomes overwhelming. We can't imagine what this weariness feels like. We've never experienced anything near it. I've heard it explained this way: imagine concrete blocks tied to every limb and you've been dragging them uphill for weeks. Somewhere along the way, you realize that you will never reach the top—it's just not to be. So you close your eyes to rest, and you're pleasantly surprised. The grass is soft and cool where you are. It is good to just lie there with your eyes closed. The sleep has relief, and the dreams are good. For the first time in a long time, you feel that maybe it's okay to not climb that hill.

"But the angst returns when you see your family, calling from the top, urging you to keep going. You can hear the distress in their voices. But you have cancer, and they don't. Even if you wanted to, you know that you can't do it anymore."

She paused, hoping that they were able to make the switch from what they were feeling to what their mother might be feeling. It would be important for their own comfort after her death. She wished that she had been able to start these conversations months ago; their bereavement would be so much easier. Sighing to herself, she pushed on.

> There's a turn the dying must make

"So my suggestion is to let her rest. And my hope for you is that you will find a way to bless her in her going, rather than asking her to remain with you.

Can you see what I'm trying to convey, Julian, even if it sounds impossible to do?"

Julian was staring down at his own hands now. A tear fell on one, and he swiped at it quickly. "I guess so," he murmured low, "but I don't like it. I want her to stay here."

The room sat in silence, honoring this young man's pain. Eventually, his sister came out of her own thoughts enough to put her arms around her brother.

"We all want her to stay, Jules. But I've had a little longer to think about it, and I can see things I didn't see before. We're going to have to let her go. The doctor's office said the cancer is really bad. Mom didn't tell us everything. I don't think she can stay here even if she wants to."

Julian tucked his head into her neck, hating that his sister was composed while he blubbered, but he was coming around to seeing that they might be right. He could see for himself that the cancer had wasted her away, but since nobody was talking about it, maybe it wouldn't actually happen … death. It seemed to be happening now, though, and his fears were almost as bad as the grief of losing her. He didn't have a family of his own like Nina had, and his mother had always been his rock. He wasn't sure how he was going to make it if she left—*when* she left.

"I don't want to do anything that makes it worse for her," he finally said to the nurse, but he was looking at Nina. "But I don't want her to die any sooner than she has to, either." This answer felt loyal—like a son should feel, looking out for his mother.

Nina kissed him on the cheek, a sisterly thing to do, he thought; then she focused her attention back on the nurse, who needed to ask a few questions as she walked them through the hospice admission process. As she ended her visit, she taped the agency phone number to the refrigerator door and encouraged them to call the nurse-line if Mrs. Rose had any changes or if they had any questions. She left, promising to be back the following day.

A Rare Rally

The next day's visit found Martina fully awake and having breakfast at the kitchen table! Nina and Julian were both present, but the girls were out for pancakes with their dad. Brother and sister were thrilled to show off their mother's improvement, and the nurse smiled broadly as she reintroduced herself to Mrs. Rose. Martina was a little fuzzy-minded, speaking in short phrases and leaving most questions unanswered. Her egg and toast sat half-eaten in front of her.

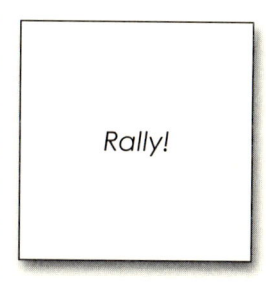

Rally!

"Mom, would you like to go back to bed now and rest?" Nina asked her. Martina nodded, and the three escorts walked her to the bedroom where she climbed into the bed by herself. She was tucked in, pillows fluffed, the light left off, and the lamp turned on by her request, a cup of coffee and a fresh glass of water on her bedside table. Having nothing left to do to love on her, Julian and Nina returned reluctantly to the living room, taking their accustomed seats. The nurse completed her assessment and soon joined them.

"Isn't this wonderful!" the nurse said warmly but then added a caution. "Enjoy these hours. They are very rare! We never know how long these rallies will last, but I'm so glad that you are getting one! It always reminds me of the 'nesting syndrome' that can happen near the end of pregnancy—a surge of energy for those last-minute details that need completing before the baby arrives."

Nina stood suddenly, interrupting her, something triggered by the pregnancy analogy. She turned sharply toward Julian.

"We have to tell Mom today that it's okay for her to leave," she said decidedly to his startled face.

Julian was taken off guard and shook his head back and forth.

"We said last night that we weren't going to do anything that might make her die sooner!" He matched her sudden intensity, distress and confusion in his eyes.

"Well, today, I've changed my mind." Nina faced him, arms

knotted. But large tears betrayed her bravado. "I feel differently about it now, Julian. That's all. Yesterday, when I realized that she really is going to die, I knew that I hadn't said some things that are important. I've felt a big hole in my heart, Jules. I don't want Mama to die trying to climb up that big hill and feeling bad about not making it." Her eyes were brimming, searching his. But Julian's hands were shoved deep into his pockets, and his foot was tapping rashly. Nina knew this stance but she pushed on.

"If I don't say my goodbyes now," she pleaded, "I'll never get the chance. So, I don't know what you're going to do, but I'm going to tell her." She didn't move, however, watching to see if her brother would be joining her or standing in her way.

Julian was so angry! His sister was taking a chance that he didn't want to take. It had been such a great surprise to see Mom awake this morning, and he just wanted to enjoy the day. Now here was his big sister, messing with it. Last night, he had also seen the image of his mom crawling up a hill with the concrete blocks, but it didn't look that way to him today. Couldn't they just leave it alone?

He stamped to the bedroom and looked in. Mom was leaning back against her pillows, peaceful, something she hadn't been in weeks. One day, yes, probably soon, he would look into that room and see an empty bed. But right now, couldn't this be good enough? It was good enough for him. How could Nina betray them by giving up on her?

He ranted internally while he stumbled back to the couch to sit down, thrusting his head into his hands, feet still drumming. He didn't make decisions quickly, like his sister seemed to.

But the picture was back, pounding in his head. What if she was right again? What if his mother was in anguish inside, because she couldn't climb the hill? Shouldn't she have some peace, even if he didn't?

Several minutes passed before he was able to look up at Nina, exhausted and exasperated. He lifted his shoulders more in acquiescence than agreement.

"Okay, I get it. We should probably try it. But it won't be mushy.

We'll just tell her that it's okay to go whenever she's ready, and that's it."

"And that we're going to be just fine on our own," Nina prompted.

He responded with a signature sibling scowl. His sister could be so pushy. Nina then turned to the nurse.

"Will you help us?"

The Children Say Goodbye

The nurse was startled by the sudden turn of events but instantly agreed.

"Of course," she nodded and then reflected a moment. "Just talk normally, and tell your mother what you're feeling. Speak slowly, and keep your sentences simple. And don't be alarmed if you don't get much reaction back," she coached. "The important thing is what she hears from you, not what she says back. She's still in a dream-state and can't think clearly. But she'll hear you. Let's see what happens."

> Saying your Good-byes

They walked together into Martina's room, the children taking seats on either edge of the bed. Martina was awake, but her eyes were closed. Her eyelids blinked open only briefly when the children called her name.

"Mom?" Nina started them out. "Can you hear me okay?"

Her mother nodded, her face working for a smile.

"Jules and I are here, and we want to tell you something. Can you listen?"

Martina nodded again, a thin but genuine smile on her lips, her eyes still closed.

Nina looked at Julian, who obviously wasn't going to be helping her out. She looked back to her mother's face and saw that the jaundice had a deep orange cast to it today.

"Mama, we know that you're tired. And ... we know that you aren't able to stay here with us." She looked up at the nurse who had taken a post at the foot of the bed. The nurse nodded her on, her eyes sad but her expression encouraging.

"Are you afraid?" Nina thought of how fearful she would be if she were the one dying.

But Martina moved her head slowly side to side, her mouth whispering, "No, not afraid. Just tired."

Nina was relieved. Julian's eyes were just staring, fixated on the fragile hand he held carefully in his own. This was no way to live, he thought, looking at the once strong hands. He looked up into Nina's eyes, nodding for her to continue. "It's okay," his eyes told her. Nina took a deep breath, feeling a peace come into her. This seemed the right thing to do. She was even able to smile a little, as she slowly spoke the words:

"Mom, Julian and I want to tell you that it's okay for you to go. We don't want you to, but we know that you have to. We're going to be brave, and we're going to be okay, and we don't want you to worry about us at all. Jules …" She looked at her brother now as she talked. "… is going to come over every night for dinner, and he's going to make sure that your granddaughters know all about you. This will be his job, to tell all his funny stories about you."

Martina's eyes remained closed, but her smile broadened. She was hearing them.

"Does this make you happy, Mama?"

"Yes, it does," she said. They thought that would be all, but Martina said more.

"I've worried about you two," she breathed. "But I know that you're going to be okay. We'll all be together again. I'm sure of it."

Julian and Nina shared a look across the bed. Mom was more alert than they had thought. Julian tried for another sentence, a happy memory to keep her smiling a little longer.

"Mom, do you remember when you took us to the beach and your hat flew off and knocked that lady's ice cream cone onto her kid's head? We laughed that whole trip. It was a great time."

Martina's lips pulled up more, but she could not hold it.

"Loved the beach," she murmured. "Love you. Sleepy."

"I love you too, Mama." Julian laid his head carefully on her chest and heard the low rattle. No, conditions had not really changed. "You get some rest. It's okay to sleep. We'll be here."

Her head gave the slightest nod, and Julian leaned over to kiss her cheek. He then rose from the bed and walked out without looking back. Nina kissed her mother's cheek also, feeling the fever returning to it.

"Her fever's back," she told the nurse when they joined Julian back in the living room.

"Yes, her temperature was 102° when I checked. And her diaper was barely wet. I was so surprised to see her awake today; I wasn't sure if it would happen. It's unusual to get the opportunity you just had. I'm so glad you were able to give her your blessing."

The kids nodded, looking at the floor, relief mixed with grief.

"You guys really did good," the nurse went on, repressing a small cheer, unable to restrain a hug for each of them. "See, you didn't need me at all. And did you see that smile? That was what she wanted, just to know that her children will be okay."

The nurse stayed a few minutes longer, answering their remaining questions and giving more instructions. Then she began making her way to the door. As she said her goodbyes, she grabbed their necks for one last hug. She had been deeply affected by what she had been invited to observe. This was why she was a hospice nurse—to be a witness to the courage of her brave families. As she closed the door behind her and headed to her next patient, Julian and Nina were left to stand alone again in the too-quiet house.

"Can you stay over for a few days?" Nina looked up at her little brother. "We can put the air mattress in Mom's room and take turns sleeping in there. I think I'm going to need some help with her."

Julian nodded, relaying that he had already taken the week off. She sent him up the street with a grocery list. Then together, they prepared one of Mom's favorite meals, hoping that she would eat again, but she didn't. Martina had fallen back into the deep sleep of yesterday, her mouth open, her breathing heavy. She slept all day, her chest rising and falling, the rattling of her throat constant.

Nina placed a few drops of medicine in her mouth as the nurse had instructed, and the rattle improved a little. She did the same with two crushed acetaminophen for the fever, but they didn't help much. Nina changed her mother's gown and her diaper. The gown was wet with sweat, but the diaper was dry.

A Journey of One

Behind the Veil

About sundown, Martina started talking, at first to her sister, who had passed before Nina and Julian were born. They sat down on either side of the bed, listening. Their mother's eyes were closed, but she was in deep chatter with someone. And laughing! She repeated the name Adela often and chuckled and smiled, as if sharing a private joke. She mentioned the name Madre also, and they wondered if this was their grandmother, who was also passed. Whatever was going on, their mother looked very happy.

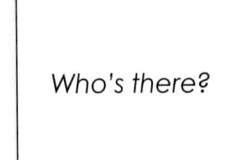

> Who's there?

"Mama? Are you talking to someone?" Nina finally asked, curious to know what was happening.

"Yes, Adela's here. She looks so pretty. And she says Madre is coming soon." Her mother's voice was calm and clear.

"Are you seeing other people too?" Julian asked, wanting to take a peek over his shoulder but resisting.

"Yes, there are more here. That's my cousin with the brown hair, and there's my old friend—I can't think of her name. I don't know some of the others." She fell silent again.

Julian spoke again. "Are you seeing a bright light?"

"No," she tilted her head a little, "it's more of a soft yellow light. Very pretty."

Julian looked over at his sister. How many more answers would they get?

"Are the people you see asking you to come with them?"

"No, they're just waiting," she said easily.

"What else do you see?" this time from Nina.

But Martina wasn't answering anymore. Her face had relaxed, and she was falling back into her deep sleep. Nina and Julian looked wide-eyed at each other. That had been amazing. Their mother was seeing people from the other side.

For two more days, Martina slept and talked; her words becoming more and more difficult to understand. If her eyes were open, they would be staring into corners or at the ceiling. And when she slept, her breathing would stop for long periods of time and then would rush to catch up. The agitation never returned. But she ate no more food and took in only the water that the kids used to keep her lips moist. The fever came and went.

Martina Makes It Home

In Martina's last hours, Nina and Julian decided not to call hospice. They were comfortable now with her care, and they wanted to have the time alone with their mother. Her breathing had softened now from deep, heavy breaths to shallow exchanges that barely lifted the sheets. She seemed comfortable, and it did not appear that there would be any more conversations or rallies. They found it peaceful to be just the three of them at the end, as it had been for most of their lives. The girls were in their room, their father supervising their quiet play.

The hospice staff had instructed and encouraged them, and they had been good learners. The social worker had helped them with funeral arrangements, and the hospice chaplain would perform a small service for them at the graveside. There was nothing else to do for the moment but to sit vigil and wait. As they waited, Julian and Nina shared quiet stories of their lives growing up. They hoped their mother could hear them.

Their mother took her last breath a little after noon. They sat holding her hands, reassuring her often that they would be okay, until there was no more need to reassure. Martina was gone.

The Last Move

It was a long time before either stirred, not wanting to leave the shelter of their mother's room. Outside was the world that demanded their attention, and now they faced it without their mother. Nina's husband finally called hospice for them and then took the girls out for ice cream. When the nurse arrived, she found Nina and Julian quietly moving about the bedroom, rearranging items that were not really out of place. They received her hugs, and she asked if they would like to be present for her last examination and preparation of their mother. They declined. Both seemed relieved to be led now, having crossed an imaginary finish line and finding themselves exhausted and numb. The two allowed themselves to be guided into the kitchen, and the nurse directed Nina to put on a pot of coffee, giving her something to do. Julian made his way to the couch and sat down heavily, leaning his head back, his arm resting over his eyes.

The nurse then returned to the bedroom, closing the door behind her. She washed Martina's body and placed a clean gown on her; then she changed the bed linens. She thought of how proud she was of these children who had pulled together so well for their mother. But it was obvious to her that they could do no more that day.

The funeral home transport team soon pulled up outside—a white SUV with a decal on the side, announcing to all that there had been a death—Martina Rose's death.

The transport lead and the nurse exchanged a few signatures, and then they disappeared into Martina's bedroom and closed the door. This was the children's first dealings with a funeral home, and they wished for a distraction. Some music or the background noise of a television set would help, but both seemed inappropriate. They sat uncomfortably on the couch instead, untouched coffee on the table in front of them, trying not to listen to the clanging and bumping noises from the other room. Eventually, the nurse slipped back out and came to sit with them.

"Okay. You've done so well, and I am very proud. You took care of your mother better than anything I have ever seen. You stuck by her and made good decisions even when it made things harder on you. This has been a very difficult road, and you've seen it through all the way to the end. Your mother would be so proud." She took the nearest hand, which was Nina's. She regarded each one of them, knowing there were still tough events ahead. But she had come to trust these two. They were steady when they were together.

"One of the hardest parts is about to come, and I want to prepare you, even though it only lasts for a few minutes." She paused, waiting until she had their full attention.

"They are going to take your mother out of the house in a moment. There is something about this that feels very final, and it can be overwhelming for some. I want you to think about where you want to be when they move the gurney out. You don't have to be here at all if you don't want to be. We can go stand in the garage or in the backyard, or we can sit right here. Wherever you would like to be."

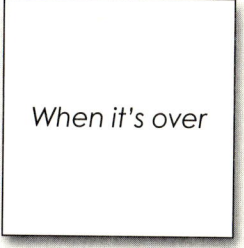

When it's over

Nina started to whimper, but Julian stood up, moving.

"I'm going to wait in the kitchen," he said, moving.

Nina blindly followed him, pale and unsteady. The nurse followed, this time taking her post near Nina, who was lowering herself to a kitchen chair.

"Are we ready?" she asked them respectfully, as the transport lead opened the bedroom door, waiting for his signal.

She paused until she had received two steady nods and then nodded her signal to the transporter. Nina moaned as the rattling of the gurney signified that their mother's body was out of the bedroom and was passing through the small living room, nearing the front door. Julian bent down and wrapped his arms around his sister, cradling her in his awkward hug. This was harder than seeing her body in the bed, he thought. He tried to hear anything but the sounds of the gurney wheels, now landing solidly on the outside walkway. They heard the SUV doors close and the crunch of gravel. Then all was quiet.

The nurse moved to take a quick turn about the bedroom, pulling up the blankets and replacing the rose that the team had laid on the pillow. She returned to the living room, where brother and sister were gratefully reclaiming their seats on the couch. There was an emptiness in the house, and they sat side by side in silence, waiting for the moment to settle. The nurse watched, familiar with the hollow vacancy that accompanied the completion of a terminal illness. All was silent until one of the children looked up at her, which she took as a signal that it was okay to speak again.

"We're not finished here," she told them, her voice feeling too loud in the stillness of the room. Julian looked up blankly; Nina only sniffled, the blood beginning to return to her face.

"Our bereavement coordinator will be in touch to see how your family is doing, and we'll continue for several months to come. We're here if you need anything, even tonight. Your mom is no longer with you, but you will be picking up the pieces and remaking a life that looks much different than what the last year has looked like. We know there are still hard days ahead—please, don't go it alone. Let us help." She paused, and they nodded, not really knowing what they were nodding to anymore.

"Will you be staying together today? Nina, is your husband off work and able to help? I'm always concerned about leaving my families after their loved one passes. What can I do for you two right now?" She watched their faces, these two beautiful young people, sitting on a faded couch, their mother dead. Some cases were just harder on the heart, and this was one of them.

"We'll be okay," Nina said, without conviction. Then she straightened her back and looked over to her brother. Her elbow nudged him gently, and she laid her head on his shoulder.

"We're going to be okay," she said again, lifting her head back. "It's been just us for a while. When Mama got sick, we had to learn how to take care of ourselves and take care of her too, so we'll figure out what to do. We're going to keep going like we've been doing, and we're going to make Mama proud, right Julian?"

He looked less sure but gave her a shrug.

"And Julian is going to tell Mama Rose stories to his nieces, and he's going to find himself a nice girl and settle down, just like Mama wanted—right, Julian?" She elbowed him again, and Julian grinned a little this time.

"I know lots of good 'Mama Rose' stories," he said, wiping at his eyes. "Especially the beach and the ice cream one. That was a good time. Maybe we can all go there this summer, in honor of Mama."

Nina smiled back and nodded a yes.

This was her cue. The nurse stood, able to let them go now. They would be all right, at least for today, and her hospice bereavement team would be following them closely. She wished their long road of grief was as easy as telling stories or going to the beach, but these were both excellent places to start. She reached over and gave them yet another hug, telling them once again how proud she was. She then turned one last time to make sure the hospice phone number was still on the refrigerator door. As she was walking out, Nina's husband was walking in, two ice cream-smeared smiles at his side.

Mrs. Martina Rose, aged forty-six, passed away peacefully at her home with family present, hospice bereavement services to follow.

QUESTIONS FOR REFLECTION
CHAPTER 4: MARTINA

1. Sleep is the single most relieving and healing experience afforded to a human being. But Martina won't sleep, so nobody is sleeping. What are some reasons that might be contributing to Martina's fear of falling asleep?

2. Nina wakes one morning to a too-quiet house and is afraid to go down the hall to check on her mother. How much does fear of seeing someone dead or dying affect your personal decision to care for a loved one during the dying process?

3. Patients often come to hospice having had many emergency room visits in which no effective treatments could be found. When Martina has a change in status, Nina must decide whether to send her again to the hospital (where Nina is most comfortable) or to remain at home where Martina is most comfortable. What feelings come up for you when you think about *not* calling an ambulance?

4. CPR (cardiopulmonary resuscitation) or DNR (do not resuscitate) is a weighty decision. CPR on television always goes well. The patient revives and sits up, and soon life returns to normal. But medical professionals know differently. What are your thoughts on "letting nature take its course" versus "use all available treatments to extend life"?

5. Telling your loved one goodbye may seem as difficult as the actual time of parting. Myriads of emotions are tied up in the thought—betrayal, giving up, letting go, it's too early, it was too late, and so on. Do you have regrets over not telling a loved one goodbye or that you loved them? Do you have other regrets that you wish you had been given time to redo? If so, how can you release yourself from this pain and be freed as your loved one is now free? (Sources suggest writing a letter, talking to your loved one as if he or she were present or holding a belated goodbye service.)

CHAPTER 5

Zoe's Journey

- Age 48, breast cancer
- Primary symptom: wound
- Primary caregivers: Jeanne and Bob

Note to the Reader

"Zoe" is a real patient, though her name and the names of her family members have been changed to protect their privacy. At the time of this writing, she still lives and lives well—not physically nor energetically but spiritually and holistically. I have included this chapter with her permission, and unlike the other chapters, which are conglomerations and combined stories of real and fabricated patients, this one has been kept true to form.

Zoe carries the worry that her cancer, her wound, and her death will be her legacy. But wait until you hear her story. I am unworthy of telling it and can only pray that her hope and her spirit and, yes, her joy, will come through in the telling. *This* is your legacy, Zoe. That you can have one of the worst cancers that this hospice nurse has ever seen and yet say that it was the best thing that ever happened to you. Your legacy is the person you have been and still are and will be to come. Thank you for allowing me to join you on your journey of one. Thank you for showing me how to journey it when it is my time.

The Road Together

Zoe

Zoe is a very busy woman. She works twelve-hour shifts as an ICU nurse, often taking overtime. She is a good nurse, actually a great nurse in the eyes of her coworkers. Zoe is conscientious, arriving early and staying late, always kind and professional, always upbeat, and always busy. She's the kind of nurse that some staff members love because she is knowledgeable and trustworthy, works hard, and always steps up to help. And others hate her because she raises the bar.

"Zoe, can't you sit down for just a minute? We're celebrating Jacquelyn's birthday party in the breakroom. Come visit for just a second. She's turning the big four-oh!"

"I'll be there in a minute," Zoe calls back from the manager's office. "I just want to check the monthly schedule again. You guys start without me."

What the others don't know is that Zoe woke at 3:00 a.m. thinking about the schedule, which she has already checked and rechecked but which caused her to throw up her morning Egg McMuffin in the parking lot anyway, an escalating habit.

Zoe? Nerves? No one would suspect. But Zoe thrives on it. Nervous energy, nervous eating, nervous sleep, overplanning, overtasking, you name it. Zoe *is* energy. She craves being pumped and adrenalized. She's always had it—higher dreams, eclectic emotions, bigger-than-life desires. And nursing was like stumbling into a new bar filled with adrenaline-junky drinking buddies. Anyone in the medical field knows the drill—long shifts, minimal sleep, understaffed, people are sick, keep it moving, can you cover the weekend shift, will you answer one more call light before you leave—and Zoe rides the wave. It's not actually nervous energy that drives her; it's really just Zoe energy. It's the "Zoe pace."

Zoe's sixteen-year-old son, Marc, is used to the Zoe pace. He doesn't subscribe to it himself. It's just not his nature. But it has wrapped itself around him and swooped him along with it since his birth. He's been raised in the world of single-motherhood but at twice the speed. He doesn't mind so much; it has its perks. He enjoys a less micromanaged school life than most of his classmates and their helicopter moms. While Zoe may not be able to buy him everything he wants, she is able to buy what he needs, plus a little extra. And Zoe loves him—he knows that and knows it very well. They have been through a lot together, he and his mother, and they are a good team. Unless she's at work, all of her attention is for him. She rouses herself from bed to attend his basketball games, cheering loudly and embarrassing him gloriously. They share the love of gory action movies and spend weekends at the movie theater and late nights watching television. His friends come over whenever they want, and if their noise is disturbing her sleep, she never lets on. Zoe is definitely not a cookie-cutter mom, and Marc loves that about her. She might not be at home as much as he wished, but all moms are like that nowadays. And the extra shifts help keep their lives going—car repairs, sports fees, the recycling of basketball shoes for his ever-growing feet, weekend money for him and a random ladies' night out for herself. They work hard, play hard, communicate by text messages and sticky notes—the usual. In Marc and Zoe's eyes, they are a typical, single-mom/teenage-boy American family.

But Zoe's body is carrying a secret. The Zoe pace is killing her. "One of these days," she tells herself, "I'm going to have to slow down, take a vacation, and drop some weight so that I don't die of a heart attack." But at forty-two, it's not a true concern. She's strong, and she's healthy, and she feels great. She has time.

The Path Bends

Diagnosed

It wasn't much of a concern to Zoe when her annual mammogram came back suspicious—15 percent of them do. And 99.5 percent of abnormal mammograms are not cancerous. But Zoe's was the fluke, and the final diagnosis *was* a shocker—not just the breast cancer itself but the aggressiveness of this cancer. A survival rate of what? How long did they say? Should I get another opinion? But everything was right there on the scan. She could see the mass and read the reports for herself. This was a devastating cancer; there was no denying it. In fact, denial was a grief stage that Zoe skipped entirely, or so she thought. But it wasn't denial of the cancer that tripped her up eventually. It was underestimating its power.

Being a nurse created a wall when it came to cancer treatments. Zoe had seen too much. Anyone who has ever attached a chemo bag to an IV pole knows that he or she is about to inject a rogue poison into a living body. Cancer cells act as if they are being controlled by an unknown alien force. Zoe and her coworkers call them "zombie cells" because they have one goal—destroy all good cells and overtake the host. Medical treatments are certainly improving, but at this time, chemotherapies are not able to target just the dangerous cells. General chemical warfare agents must be pumped into the bloodstream with the hope that the hungry cancer cells will drink up more than the normal cells will and that too many normal cells will not be killed in the process.

Unfortunately, there are civilian casualties in any war, and normal cells die in this battle as well—brain cells, muscle cells, blood vessels, stomach lining, liver cells, lung cells, and the list goes on. And then a barrage of radiation treatments usually follows, causing further mayhem.

"And it's such overkill!" Zoe jokes irreverently to a friend at the hospital lockers, where she has been stopped to give an account of her last oncology appointment.

"Yes, it is definitely cancer, but I'm feeling great," Zoe beams characteristically. "It's something I'm going to have to deal with for sure, but I've already missed too much work for doctor's appointments, and I can't miss any more right now." She turns breezily to her

> *The 5 Stages of Grief:*
> *denial*
> *anger*
> *bargaining*
> *depression*
> *acceptance*

locker, missing the dagger eyebrows launched at her back. Does Zoe not understand her diagnosis? And she's thinking of delaying chemo and radiation? Surely that's a death sentence! But her friend holds her tongue.

"So, what's your next step then? Surgery?" she probes.

"I've already talked with a surgeon about it," Zoe throws over her shoulder. "I'd like to have the tumor removed, but the surgeon said that if he were to accidentally cut through the margins, which he can't always avoid, then it might cause the cancer to spread. And if I won't take the chemotherapy to kill what gets spread, then it puts his office at too much risk. He said that I could 'sue his suspenders off.'" She laughs, turning and stretching out imaginary suspenders. "Which I would never do, of course. But he refused the surgery anyway. I'll get another opinion, but I bet I get the same answer. It makes sense from a lawyer's point of view, but it sure leaves me facing a wall."

"Wow," her friend frowns, her voice taut. "So you're going to have a growing tumor in your breast that you won't kill and you can't get cut out either. So tell me your plan again, Zoe? You're going to just let it fall off?"

Zoe takes no offense to the wisecrack. This is just nurse jargon for "I care about you, and what are we going to do to fix this problem?"

"I'm going holistic."

"Holistic!" the nurse shrills, too loud for the small room. "Zoe, you can't be serious! Eating green beans instead of ice cream does not cure cancer! You've got to have a better plan than this. At least get some more opinions or something." Her sarcasm does have real concern. This is her friend, her coworker, and everyone else's cheerleader. She is planning to aim a pea shooter at a giant, and she is going to lose. Maybe this is denial? It is bargaining at the very least. Zoe's crazy plan is to substitute celery for silver bullets.

"I can't stand by and watch you do this, Zoe. We've got to talk more. Call me, okay? I'll listen, but I am going to try to talk you out of this. I care too much about you to see you throw your life away.

And you've got Marc to think about. Your responsibility is to do everything you can to stay alive!" The nurse paced the small room now, three steps one way, three steps return.

"This really has me upset!" Her hands gesture as she turns again. "I'm sorry, but I just can't believe what you're telling me. Please, Zoe, change your mind before this thing grows too big. Please. Just think about it. And call me. We'll talk." She makes a last turn and paces out, presumably to tell every coworker from here to the front door that Zoe has lost her mind and is going to use tree nuts to cure her cancer.

Zoe's Choice

But Zoe has seen too many cancer treatment disasters, and she knows she has to find another way. Standing at the locker, her mind reviews the line-up—the patient who came in for radiation on his chest and ended up with a melted trachea and esophagus, the chemotherapy IV that infiltrated and resulted in a lost arm, the woman who walked in for treatment and was rolled out the back on a gurney. Too many stories, too many horrors. There are good stories too, of course—Mr. Charles, who comes in every few months to bring them chocolates and to thank them for helping him survive, Mrs. Kennedy who was pregnant when diagnosed with uterine cancer and brings her son to their floor on his birthdays. But those seem to be the rare ones. Or maybe it is just that she works in a hospital so is more likely to be present for the scenarios that go badly. Whatever the reasons, Zoe has seen too many people walk in healthy for their first chemo appointments and then be wheeled out weak and half-dead by their last treatment. She cannot do it that way—not as a single mother, not as a full-of-life young woman, not as a nurse.

A first moment of fear seeps into the still locker room. Zoe leans her head against the cool metal, allowing the moment. Is she in denial? Does she really believe that those were *her* scans on that monitor? Has she honestly accepted that there is a tumor growing and killing inside her? But, surely, a single mother with a son to raise would not be asked to go through this. Surely, God will find her a better way. She will research her options this weekend, next week at the very latest. Zoe, God, and the strong body He has given her will sort this out, somehow. In the meantime, life calls, so Zoe answers, characteristically.

Holistic Roadblocks

Zoe didn't know very much about holistic medicine when she started. For her, the name conjured up stories of trips to exotic lands for magic miracle cures. She found a few local medical offices that offered holistic therapies but met another wall when she was told that all payments would need to be out-of-pocket.

> Alternative medicine and insurance

Zoe has excellent medical insurance, but it is useless unless she takes the traditional medical routes "as prescribed." And traditional routes are generally all or nothing: you cannot pick and choose your own therapies. Well, she grants wryly, that is not entirely true. You *can* choose to decline a treatment, like radiation or chemotherapy, but you find herself labeled "noncompliant" and blocked from the system almost entirely, as she had found with the surgeon. And *that* became the final wall that locked Zoe in.

She continued to work; continued to shop, cook, and clean; continued attending basketball games and sharing late-night TV with Marc. On her days off, she dug through the internet and crossed swords with medical and insurance entities. She could feel no lump and had no pain, but she was aware of a growing tug at the outside of her right breast when she lifted groceries or reached across for her seat belt. Nothing much, only a tug. But it was there.

> Holistic: physical

Zoe's internet research took her to several cancer treatment sites in South America and Mexico, and she found herself dreaming of sipping flavored cancer tonics on a restful beach. She thought seriously about this option and researched it thoroughly. The centers offered treatments available now, which the more conservative US agencies would not approve for many years to come, if at all. Prior to her own diagnosis, she had been all for the more diligent regulations. But now ... well, let's just say that Mexico was very tempting, but not very practical, she finally decided. The internet reviews were too mixed. In the end, she decided to buy some of their products—phytonutrients and aloe vera mixes—and sit in her own backyard to drink them, imagining the beach. That, she declared, was something she *could* do.

The most productive piece of information that Zoe learned from her research is that cancer can be caused and worsened by inflammation of any sort. Stress, anxiety, trauma, unhealthy diet, poor sleep, exposure to toxins—all are agents of inflammation. In order for a holistic approach to work, she would have to completely eliminate all inflammation sources from every aspect of her life.

Hospice Admission

"It's called 'holistic' because every mind and body system must be on board, or it won't work. And that's where I messed up." Zoe shares this matter-of-factly at our hospice admission, now sixteen months since her cancer diagnosis. We sit in a sunny front parlor, where Zoe and her mother, Jeanne, spend much of their day. An elderly golden retriever and a rescued German shepherd lay at our feet. Jeanne has offered tea with honey, and sitting in the sunny parlor, I find myself bonding immediately with this family. Zoe and I have worked out that we started our careers at the same hospital, though in different eras. And earlier in my years, I had lived a "Zoe pace" as well, so I understood intimately the joys and disasters of it. "And," I share as I sip the delicious tea, "we are practically neighbors." My new home is only a few miles down the road.

Commonalities aside, these are easy people to love on their own merit. There is a presence in this home that I rarely find in terminally ill environments. I come across it mostly in elderly couples who know—just inexplicably know—that the road will continue on "until one lays the other in the arms of God" and that they will be rejoined later.

I also have no doubt by the present conversation that is unwrapping that the opportunity for friction in this home is certainly available as well. Zoe calmly relays the year of contending with the obstinate medical system, one which she loves and ultimately still respects. Jeanne speaks quietly of wanting to support her daughter but not knowing how, believing that she was on a hopeless path. Both women, sitting in different life-and-death viewpoints, are genuine, somehow able to truly love and support the other. I marvel. Both lives have been altered because of Zoe's decisions, no doubt. Zoe has been forced to move herself and Marc into her parents' home. Along with the general effort of managing the household, Jeanne preps Zoe's fresh-food-only regimen, which requires an enormous amount of kitchen time. Zoe's parents are more than happy to accommodate, and they love having Zoe and Marc with them. But it does create hardships, both physically and emotionally. And there is no getting around the fact that Zoe's plan has not worked as hoped. True, it is also very possible that the traditional route of cancer treatments would have brought them to this same point. Regardless, hospice is now here, marking the beginning of the end of the journey. It hangs in the air over our admission paperwork, though we all discreetly ignore it.

The Best Thing That Ever Happened

Hospice visits are established for Zoe, and we eventually develop a routine. At this particular visit, Zoe and I stand in her small bathroom performing the weekly measuring of her tumor, officially labeled "wound" in my chart. I have to say that it is quite an impressive one. Every measurement shows the tumor inching further in every direction—spreading wider, bubbling up at the edges, cratering in at the center. The surface of the wound is roughly the size of my hand. Zoe manages it well, her composure in check, her countenance calm. She changes the outer dressing several times both day and night because of the large amount of drainage that soaks quickly through the thick dressing pads. The inner dressings are of a special medicated material that are designed to be changed weekly, but after forty-eight hours, they are saturated and pungent. Zoe and I talk as we work, mostly out of friendship but also to counter the awkwardness of two people standing in a tiny bathroom, padding and taping a breast.

"Tell me what your life was like just before hospice was called in," I ask, to jump-start a conversation. Zoe is happy to share. She has dealt phenomenally with the diagnosis, the decisions, the walls and the fall-out, but that doesn't mean she isn't appreciative of a sympathetic ear.

"By the time I genuinely understood what a holistic approach meant and had learned how to get all systems on board," she tells me pragmatically, "it was basically too late." Her words are simple statements, neither protective nor controlled. I hear hints of regret but little resentment, which is Zoe's way.

"My cancer had grown and spread too far to warrant asking for treatment even if I wanted it, which I'm still not sure that I do." Zoe looks at me untroubled, not as I expect a young woman with terminal cancer to be.

"Explain more about all systems needing to be on board," I pry, working at a section of tape that stretches from sternum to mid-back. I have never known anyone who has carried a holistic approach this far, and I am a listener, for as long as she will talk. I stand at her right side while she uses the bathroom mirror to point and hand me dressings. She is much more adept at this than I, and we both know that she is only being polite, letting me be the nurse for the visit so that I can feel useful. I have finally pulled away the old tape and am busy tearing thin strips off the new roll.

"Leigh," Zoe abruptly turns my way, stopping my work. "I'm not sick because I have cancer; I have cancer because I am sick."

I straighten to look at her face, not understanding. Lengths of tape dangle from my gloved fingers. For the first real time, I see Zoe's face pinch with tension and pain. She has something to say.

"I was a very sick person, but I didn't know it. Actually, I guess we're all aware when something is wrong, but as long as we can keep going, we will. And the problem just gets shoved aside for another day. But physical health is not stagnant. Mental health isn't either. You're either getting better or you're getting bitter, and, girl, I was bitter. Even I didn't know how bitter I was, because I just kept smiling and pushing through it. But holistic health means that your body, your mind, your emotions, and your spirit are *all* working together for healing.

"Keep talking. You've got my attention," I say, ignoring the tape strips grabbing for each other during my inattentiveness. Gloves and tape just do not mix. Zoe is facing me straight on, the half-covered wound out of my reach, her over-sized shirt pulled up high over her shoulder. A breast becomes like a knee or an elbow after you've had to expose it repeatedly. And except for the uneasiness on her face, Zoe converses as if we are having coffee at a favorite restaurant.

"It makes sense that certain foods cause damage to your body, right? High fructose corn syrup, cheeses that don't melt after years on the counter, gluten, dairy, Twinkies—you know the list." I nod yes, I know the list. But I am offended that she has disrespected the Twinkie—I grew up on those.

"Well, being angry with someone also causes damage. It releases cortisol, which is even nicknamed the stress hormone. I've been angry at things like traffic jams, work schedules, and especially my ex, for two decades now. I tried to ignore it, but instead of clearing it all from my heart, I kept it there, adding layer upon layer of damage to my emotional system. Isn't it funny that we even have a phrase, 'It is eating me alive'? We're talking about an emotion, but doesn't that sound like cancer?"

Wow, I have to agree that it does.

"So with everything else going on, you had to learn how not to be angry?" This is astounding to me. I am more than curious to know if she had managed it. This would be a special person indeed, though I already know that this is what is standing in front of me.

"I think that not getting angry is impossible. The anger comes because we're human, and we have emotions and triggers. But did you know that an emotion only lasts for ninety seconds? A chemical gets released and floats around your system for just ninety seconds; then it's gone. But if we *want* the feeling to remain, then we hang on to the aftereffect of the feeling. Or maybe we just hit the anger button over and over, like a pain pump. You get a hit, it feels good, so you push the button again. Anger is an energy, and I was using it for fuel. I was super-nurse, supermom, super-happy ... but also super-sad and super-afraid. As long as I kept busy, I didn't have to feel. And I didn't have to get help. I could make money instead of spending money on a therapist. I could buy guilt gifts and things for Marc since I felt bad about leaving him alone so much ..."

> Holistic: emotional

She stops in mid-sentence, her lips pressed, shoulders tight. I watch her as she stares into a corner of the bathroom ceiling, remembering and feeling. But I gauge that she is also working at something else—she is releasing it. It takes several minutes, two women standing silently in a quiet bathroom, but she accomplishes it.

"I remember, and I feel terrible about it. And now I have cancer, and I have no idea if I made the right decision or not. If I had been able to stop my life and get the help that I really needed—therapy, divorce recovery, meditation classes, spiritual help, diet classes, time to just sleep and heal—maybe I could have beaten this thing. Or if I had taken the cancer treatments, I might have lived longer and even snagged a full remission. But I still believe that I chose the right way. Mostly because those other paths were solely for the purpose of living longer. I don't think that's the goal for me now. You can't know how I hate to leave Marc; I can't even conceive of it. I feel guilty, I feel angry, I feel helpless. He is the most important thing to me, my only love, and I have failed him." Her eyes well over this time, spilling tears onto her half-dressed wound. "Most people just get hypertension or a stomach ulcer when they overstress. I got cancer. It's not right, and it's not fair, but ..."

The half-taped dressing loosens, drooping and exposing. I reach with my free hand to grab at it, but she brushes my hand away. She doesn't want covering, she wants ... what? Justice? Validation? Maybe just to be heard. Zoe has an important message for me to hear. She anchors her hands solidly onto my shoulders, her eyes overflowing and compelling, her spirit full of her conviction. I have no doubt that what she is about to say is a critical statement, worthy of all my attention. I stop my attempts to catch the dressing and look her in the eyes, fully present.

"This cancer is the best thing that ever happened to me."

Did I hear her right? A young woman in her prime, a son, a career, and a life, a family who is going to be devastated, and a disfiguring wound that will eventually kill her, and she is grateful for this?

"Tell me again, Zoe," I say. "I think I misheard you."

She laughs her Zoe-laugh, releasing my shoulders and turning back to the mirror. She deftly repositions the dressing and pulls a single untangled piece of tape from my glove.

"I know. It's the strangest thing I've ever thought too. But it's true. My body was well, but now it's sick, but my soul was sick, and now it is well. It's the better swap. Go figure."

I find myself suddenly wanting to know everything that Zoe knows.

Zoe and God

Four months later finds the three of us enjoying tea again in Jeanne's comfortable parlor, a warm muzzle resting on my foot. The dogs have taken to me, and I love them (despite being a cat person in my soul of souls). My visit is complete, and my paperwork is signed off,

Holistic: spiritual

but the two ladies seem happy to keep me there for company, and I am enjoying the "professional yet friends" relationship myself. We have covered the physical and the emotional aspects of Zoe's well-being during the visit, and I am curious now about what she feels about the God who has allowed her cancer. So I question.

"Zoe, what kind of faith do you have?"

Zoe sips on tea also, but hers is spiked with bitter essential oils. I am grateful to have just sweet honey in mine.

"I still go to the same church whenever I can get there," she muses, "but something inside me has changed. I used to just attend and try to make it work, but for some reason, things make sense now. The church didn't change a bit; it was me. Something inside *me* changed. It wasn't anything I made happen or even knew to ask for. It just *changed* when I could no longer fight life, and I had to give it up. Then it happened, just like that. You'd think that letting go of it all would make you feel defeated, but it didn't. It just made me feel—I don't know—relaxed. Like floating on a raft in the ocean because your ship sailed off. You can kick and yell and scream and worry yourself to death on your raft if you want, but eventually, you just have to give up and lie down and float there! It's simpler than you think. Of course, I wish that I could have found this out earlier, without having cancer to beat it out of me, but I don't think I was capable. I believe I would have lived the same stressed-out, throwing-up, full-but-unfulfilled life for another twenty years and then would have just keeled over from a heart attack. But now I have 'a peace that passeth understanding' is the only way I know to describe it. I'm content for the first time in my life. Isn't it bizarre? Cancer made me happy."

And I believe her. It enters my mind that medications could be contributing to the effect, but I discard the thought. I have seen a drug-induced "peace that passeth understanding" many times before, and this is different. Besides, Zoe rarely takes medications. She is not opposed to them, but they are "stealers" rather than "builders" in her holistic approach, so she uses them sparingly.

The topic meanders on to other things: Marc and the start of his senior year, the hope for a weather change, the best place to buy fresh seasonal foods—normal things. But I note decline markers as Zoe talks. She is down forty pounds, which she attributes for the most part to the healthy diet. But she has also become unable to tolerate certain foods. Nausea and stomach pains are a new issue, and we have lately tweaked medications and discussed diet approaches, weighing the options of eating for comfort versus eating for nutrition. And, foreseen but unsolvable, Zoe's savings are depleted. Her semiretired parents are now covering her and Marc's expenses, and finances are tight.

Most regrettable, though, is that the cancer that induced Zoe to create her intensive holistic offensive is now forcing a retreat. The South American supplements and tonics are expensive, and the tumor continues to grow, so together the family has made the difficult decision to discontinue them. Zoe relies only on good clean foods and local supplements now. The countenance and peace of the family still prevails, and there is no mistaking that Zoe is living better at this time than she ever has before. I glance over to Jeanne, sitting comfortably in a muted yellow chair, her legs tucked gracefully underneath her. She listens to our conversation, nodding when appropriate but chiming in little. Her eyes are mist-filled, but her smile is all-in.

Jeanne's care is what makes Zoe's life work, and that is saying everything. When you choose a narrow path rather than the paved freeway of tradition, few know how to follow you. Jeanne had not believed in Zoe's choices for treatment, but she does believe in Zoe. After digging up every bit of information she could find, she had apparently spelled out her full and complete opposition to her daughter's treatment plan. But when the final decision was made, Jeanne joined in, bravely picking up her backpack to follow Zoe down the uncharted path.

"I don't know what it looks like, but I'll help you get there," became Jeanne's banner of love, and the comrades-in-arms support has been beautiful for both but especially for Zoe, as she tells me every visit. Jeanne does the shopping, the chopping, the juicing, the measuring and weighing, the cleaning of the dishes, and the managing of the double household. And Zoe's eyes brim every time she speaks of her father. Bob provides the finances, the repairs, the strong shoulder to cry on, and the care of Marc, keeping him tucked in close and answering the hard questions as they come. Marc is nearly eighteen now, his birth-father loving but not good in crisis and his mother with cancer. In fact, I speculate to myself, Bob may have the most difficult job of them all.

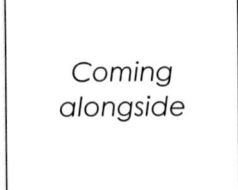

> *Coming alongside*

The Crossroads

A Troublesome Visit

Today's visit is a little more worrisome, starting with Zoe requesting that I see her in her bedroom instead of in the front parlor. Jeanne lets me in, and I follow Zoe's voice through the parlor and back to her small bedroom. The house is an old house, relocated from a historic part of town, and it has "good bones," as they say. Zoe's bedroom has high ceilings and is furnished with a large dresser and a queen-sized bed. The coverlet is a soft sage that matches the wall color. There is a nice warmth to the room, and a soft light hovers over the bed, created by a silk shade that ornaments the old wood-framed window. I take the time to describe this room because Zoe is spending more time in it now. Quite possibly, she will die in this room, she points out to me as she waves me to sit down opposite her on the coverlet. Our conversations flow easily like this now. Anything is safe to say. I ask her how she feels about dying in the room, and she says that she doesn't mind it. She's always loved this little room. She likes looking at the pictures and the knickknacks, remembering when she got them and what they mean. Zoe appears a little dreamy-minded this visit, and I inquire about her pain medicines. She tells me she took one about an hour ago and that it might have been too strong, because she feels a little drowsy now. But she also reports that she's been unusually tired for several days now.

"I'm not ready to die yet," she tells me flatly, directly. I wince. I don't want her to die either. I'm hoping this might be something else besides disease progression. With school back in session, all sorts of viruses and such are going around, and I mention it to her.

"That's true—thank you for that!" She has pushed herself up against the wooden headboard and smiles broadly at me. Such a little thing, hope. But we also both know that she should have thought of this on her own but hadn't.

Zoe answers my assessment questions and updates me on her physical status—her pain scale, fatigue scale, anxiety scale, sleep scale, bowel movements, and so on. I count her medicines and supplies and order an additional supply of dressing material. The growing wound has a bit of an odor to it now. I also request an increase in hydrocodone, as Zoe is taking it regularly now, the wound tugging and pulling, digging and deepening.

Still in assessment mode, I drill Zoe about her pain management.

"Zoe, are you taking the morphine liquid when you need it? It starts working immediately and will help with the sharp pains you have. Or you can take it before your bath or dressing changes. Just make sure someone is here with you. Once you get past the bitter taste, most patients say it works very well."

"I've used it a few times, but I don't really need it yet," she tells me. Then her voice drops, the next sentence so soft that I have to lean in to hear her.

"A few days ago, I showed my mother how to give it to me." I didn't catch her meaning. Didn't all caregivers know how to give patient medications?

"In case something happens to me," she goes on. "I keep thinking, if this tumor is growing so big on the outside, what is it doing on the inside? I don't want something horrible to happen, and I'm in pain, and no one knows how to give me the pain medicine."

I felt terrible. I always teach the caregivers how to give the medicines but had somehow assumed along the way that Zoe had been sharing all the medical information with her mother. But mothers were mothers first, not "caregivers." I would need to be more vigilant for Zoe.

"I've also been asking her to sleep in my bed with me at night, at least until I fall asleep. Is that too weird? It just makes me feel safe, and I want her close right now. I guess I'm getting mushy." Zoe's smile is tired, sad. She is definitely mushy, but it is a good look on her, and I tell her so.

"Zoe," I decide to broach, "do you want to talk about the end? It's early, but I'm here for that when you want to talk about it."

She is quiet, and I worry that I've said too much.

"I'm still afraid of it, but tell me a little bit. Just something simple." She scoots back down and lays against her pillow. I find myself leaning back against the headboard. Just girl talk here, nothing foreboding or scary.

"Okay," I say, wondering what to pick and choose. Zoe knows the physical changes that will happen, being a hospital nurse. But being a hospice nurse, I have seen some things that I am pretty sure she has not.

Jake and Gladys

"Have I ever told you the story about Jake and Gladys?"

"No," she smiles, actually snuggling down into her covers. Yes, mushy looks good on her. It makes me smile, and I shift down a bit too.

"Years ago, I was sent to a home admission for a ninety-seven-year-old gentleman. As I walked into his room, I saw immediately that I would be doing ... well, a death visit, as well as an admission visit." Dear me, I am not starting this well. But she keeps a straight face and does not flinch. Like I've said, Zoe is a good nurse.

"I was sitting beside him, watching and charting. His breathing was labored, and his oxygen levels were dropping even as I sat. I figured he had a couple of hours at best. All of a sudden, this gentleman sits straight up in bed, his eyes pop open, and he throws his arm up above his head, snapping his fingers!

"'Gladys?' he yells like a bullhorn, looking right through me.

"'Yeah, Jake?' I hear a return call from a room somewhere behind me.

"'Have you called that preacher yet to tell him I'm dying?'

"'No, Jake, I haven't done that yet.'

"'Well, you'd better. I'm not going to be here much longer.' And Jake falls back against his pillows. Immediately, his breathing is deep and heavy again. Well, I'm stunned! This man is obviously dying soon, yet he sounds like a thirty-year-old making a to-do list! There is no fear, no anxiety, no worry at all. Just facts and statements as if he were going out to the garage to get a wrench. You can imagine that I marveled at what it might mean. Apparently, Zoe, our minds don't close down and go away like I assumed. By the look of him, his mind should be cloudy and confused or gone completely—but it wasn't! At least not in his world."

"Zoe," I turn, looking straight across the pillows at her. Her lids are drooping, but she is listening. "I've come to believe that our 'mind,' or our 'soul' or whoever we really are when this tent falls apart, doesn't change a bit. I don't think that the person dying even has the experience of dying! I've seen enough in my hospice years to believe that we just change forms and keep on going."

"I think that too," she tells me with closed eyes. "Especially lately. I think God has given me a reassurance about it. I can't say why. I just kind of 'know' it, you know? So what happened to old Jake?"

"Well, Jake fell back to sleep, then a half-hour later, he did it again! Same conversation. But this time, he was more adamant about not being here much longer. And sure enough, he passed away a few hours later." I stop short, looking over to see if my ending has been inappropriate.

But Zoe just asks sleepily, "What happened to the preacher?"

I grin. I didn't usually include the encore, but it really is the best part.

"Well," I lean back, smiling and remembering. "After the second episode, I just have to go find Gladys. So I wind my way back to the kitchen. 'Gladys,' I tell her, 'Mr. Jake really isn't going to be here much longer. Don't you think you should call that preacher?' She looks at me straight-faced, doesn't even pull her hands out of the dishwater. 'Oh, darlin', his preacher died ten years ago. He doesn't even like the new one.'"

Zoe busts out a laugh, telling me I'm lying. I declare it solid truth, and we both roll hysterically, throwing around something about life being funnier than fiction. Little moments of grace.

A Journey of One

My Last Visit with Zoe

As of this writing, Zoe continues with good days and bad days. She has had weeks of pure rally, feeling great and accompanying her mother to the grocery, attending Marc's school events, and needing few pain pills. But her tumor still grows. In fact, I am taken aback by the fierceness of the thing. It is now the size of two hands.

But Zoe and I talk about more important things now—Marc's new school, the adjustment difficulties that he is working through, his new car. I see the wistfulness and the ache that she can't always be there for him. "But I have cancer," she says quietly, "and some decisions have been made for me. We all have to accept them."

I nod, feeling a recurring old anger rise in me regarding a disease that takes parents and leaves families. But I too must let it go, learning my lessons from Zoe.

"Leigh," Zoe calls me out of my reverie. She is thinner, paler, but every bit still Zoe. "I'm ready to die now." She looks over at me from her chair, and I stare back, eyebrows raised, waiting for the punch line.

"I don't mean today, but whenever it comes. I've been having these dreams lately, and they're good ones. I almost look forward to going to sleep, because I feel better in my dreams, and I feel so tired here. Is that wrong? But it's like I can't help it. I'm just kind of ready for it to be over. I don't want my family to know that; they won't understand. But every moment here is hard. This thing on my breast always tugs and pulls and drains and smells. And getting up from my chair and walking to the bathroom is hard to even think about. I don't really want to eat, even though Mom has worked so hard." She stops for a minute, catching her breath.

"I can't read Marc completely," she goes on. "You know how wonderfully mysterious boys are. He's staying close, but he looks afraid to me. No one knows what to say to me, and I don't have any energy to make them feel comfortable. None of us really *wants* it to end, of course, but we kind of need it to. They're going to go on with their lives anyway—what's a few extra weeks or whatever? And I feel like I'm going on to live too. It doesn't feel like 'dying' per se. More like slipping into a sleep that I can't stay awake from. But even that feels friendly, not fearful. Does any of this make sense? Am I talking crazy?"

You and a lot of other fully sane people in your shoes, I think to myself. But I restrain the comment.

"Sounds to me like you're doing it just right, Zoe," I try to assure her. "You're maintaining the part that you can, and everyone else is prepared that your participation will become less and less. So you just think about what you need in a day and be okay with that. You've had all the conversations that you want to have? You've said early goodbyes and have given them all permission to go on with their lives? You've resolved any regrets and have made amends?"

Zoe nods solidly as I run through the list of what is most grieved in bereavement sessions.

"I don't know what else you can do then."

We sit in a comfortable silence for a bit, me pondering, Zoe smiling. I glance at her and then close my eyes, wondering what it's like to be Zoe—contemplating what she's smiling about. Then it hits me.

"You know what, Zoe?" I sit up, declaring the profound. "Your holistic plan has worked after all! You have become whole in mind, spirit, and emotions. The last puzzle piece is in body, and when it's time, that wholeness is coming too!"

She just grins her big Zoe smile at me. Zoe has known this for a while.

Zoe, aged forty-four, lives at peace with her family, happy and whole. She sends her blessings and best wishes.

QUESTIONS FOR REFLECTION
CHAPTER 5: ZOE

1. As a nurse, Zoe had seen how cancer treatments can steal life from a person just as surely as the cancer itself can. Some people are cured by conventional treatments, and some are not. Some people are cured by holistic treatments, and some are not. Both have their risks and disadvantages. Neither has a sure outcome. Do you have strong views one way or another? How do you handle others who believe just as strongly in another view?

2. Zoe spends a lot of time explaining that all systems needed to be on board in order for her body to function freely enough to heal a deadly cancer. Poor diet, cigarettes, alcohol, and so on are known carcinogens. But do you believe that anger, fear, stress, and unresolved issues can create a toxic environment in you? What about spiritual issues—can they be toxic as well as healing? If you had to rate yourself in the areas of physical, emotional, and spiritual health, where would you fall? (Some sources also include intellectual and social areas.)

3. Zoe's family is close, supportive, and loving. In fact, Zoe and her family would like to share with you that there were times when they loved Zoe too much! But with help, Zoe's family learned better coping skills. Have you experienced a similar situation in which your relationship with a loved one was "too close"?

4. Zoe tells us that her greatest fear and loss is the thought of leaving her son. But Zoe will also leave Marc with the legacy of her spirit and her faith. Zoe really did say, "Cancer made me happy." Not always, and not every day, but through her cancer, Zoe found a happiness and peace. She found God and reconciled with Him. Reconciled means "the end of the estrangement." Have you reconciled? Are you at the "end of your estrangement" with God?

5. Like all of us, Zoe's time line is unknown. It is said that once you hear the word cancer your life is never the same. Those of us who have never heard the word cannot truly know what this is like. Take some time and reflect on someone you know who has survived cancer. What might he or she know about life that you don't know but would like to?

CHAPTER

6

The "Loved One"

Dream Vision: What It's Like for Me

Note to the Reader

What really happens on the other side is ultimately unknowable, but there are some who have touched the entrance doors. One skill of a good listener is having the ability to place yourself into a story, feeling and experiencing it from within. I am a good listener, and I have been at the side of many dying patients. They are the real storytellers here. This is a weaving of their journeys, illustrated by the story of a shop owner who finds himself dying. The purpose of this story is to aid us in visualizing what it might be like for our loved one, as he or she slips away from us and passes into the next life.

~What *we* are seeing is not what *they* are experiencing.~

What It Is Like for Me

I am the owner of a small specialty store, one that I have lived and worked in since my birth and of which I have only recently become the full proprietor, knowing where every item is located and how to best manage this singular and unique propriety. Though I have always been the owner of this business, others have often been involved with its management, especially during the early years of my training. It is a difficult thing, to manage such a distinct property. It has always been a solid structure, well-built and strong, busy in its purposes. It holds a steady position in the neighborhood, adored by some, enjoyed by others, and simply well-known and comforting to bystanders who are familiar with its presence among them. I, myself, am just learning to enjoy the entirety of the shop and its hard-fought acceptance in the community.

But, quite unexpectedly and against my will, my beloved shop is apparently to be closed down. The explanation for this has been given me, but I am at odds as to what can be done about it. The decision, and indeed the disassembling of the shop itself, seems to have been taken from of my hands, even though I am owner and manager. I so desire to keep my little shop open. I have sought all manner of fortification, but someone or something—movers or deconstruction workers, I suppose—has been at work behind the scenes. Things are strangely missing and misplaced. I have found my shop to be in such disarray of late. It is ceasing to be the well-run companion that I have known for these many years.

Fortunately, most of the meddling appears to be among items that are stored in the back, where no one yet notices. Shelves and boxes have been rifled, I can tell, and I suspect that a few items have been completely removed. As a small example, I know I had a box of delicious desserts that I was savoring, but my desire to eat them has been mislaid by these underhanded bandits. As I move my hand to my face and cheekbones, I feel the price of the misfiled appetite. I am fairly sure that no one else has noticed, but I do not know how much longer I can keep my secret.

Today, as I awoke and took inventory, I was alarmed to find several thefts on the more forward shelves, and I believe that some of my visitors may have noticed as well. Eyes widen a little, but they are gracious to display broad smiles, their voices pitching high and energetic, a pretense for my benefit. I am grateful but am chagrined. I have been such a proud owner, powering around in my shop as if it would last forever, and now it is showing signs of a destined failure.

Failure? That is an odd word to use, because all businesses eventually close or move on, don't they? But "failure" is what it appears like. It is so sad that my mind feels young and still has many plans. But I am fully aware now that these plans must change—they are simply not to be. I wonder if I am understanding a thing that my clientele does not yet accept, that my shop is moving. Or is it possible that they have known before me? It is a conversation that we do not have.

Further days of disassembling and extrication come and go. By now, I am assured that everyone can see the changes in the little shop. I note the deferential faces that my visitors wear for me, careful not to stare at the decorations that hang loosely from walls, the previously well-stocked cubbies that are now gutted. I am appreciative of this dance of disguise that we share, but at times, I would like to end the charade. It is a strange thing. My shop is truly approaching its closing date, but nobody talks about it.

I am often tired now, and I wonder if I should speak of it. The time goes by so quickly—and yet not. I do not want to worry my loved ones about the store—our store—and its inevitable demise. They have been so hopeful that it would somehow be rescued. I was as well. But I am settled with the knowledge now, as if it has been written on the shop wall.

I wonder what I will do next? I have been a shop owner all of my life. I assume that something will be arranged for me. Or possibly it will not. I suppose that I will find out when the time comes.

This is another peculiar thing, that I am not as worried as I should be. Panic and fear should be my companions, yes? My store is near closing—my life is ending! But I feel neither of these emotions. Maybe they have also been junked by the movers?

Or perhaps, perhaps, it is the latest bandit in my store. This one comes most often in the evenings, when my guard is down. I can't say that this bandit is comforting, but comfort does seem to follow behind him.

I will call him the "Dismantler." He is, it appears, a more specialized mover, the handler of personal and delicate items. He has apparently come to disassemble the store owner himself: the master, the mind, the "me." I have worked to ignore his persistent tinkerings, but am unable to keep an eye on him when I sleep or rest my eyes, as I am prone to do more often these days. When I wake, he is often standing very near, and I can tell that he has been working—surreptitiously but with alarming efficiency. I feel him step away as I pull myself up from my deepening sleeps, but he remains longer and nearer with each day. If he is the one responsible for the blurring of my fear and worry, then I suppose I am grateful for him. But he is also not judicious as to which feelings he dulls. No, that is not correct. He dismembers not the feeling itself but the adjoining connectors. A thought approaches, but its purpose and network soon dissolves, and the whole falls away. Inexplicably, I find this freeing, relaxing, calming. But he is indiscriminate. Other feelings—memories, them, me—also fall to his chopping block. I cannot remember things, important and internal things, connections that belong to my very soul. I am occasionally hit with heart-wrench at this loss. But even this upset will disassemble soon.

I require sleep. My connectors are mere gossamer strands now, and the heaviness of my eyelids is overpowering, relentless. The Dismantler has grown bold, now working into my afternoons and early mornings. I have some clarity during bright daylight, but otherwise, I am drifting, floating. Dreaming? Or not. Is it the Dismantler, or has he brought in yet another specialist, while I am incapacitated and unable to guard my watchtowers. I should be angry about this, but it does not stick. In fact, I must actually commend this work crew. There is an order here that was not understood at first. There is a method and a timing that overlaps and overlays, and it is a perfection. I am glad now that this was not left to me to accomplish, as I would have painfully botched it. This crew has dismantled and moved many a storefront—this, I can tell. My query, of which I cannot retain memory nor long concern, is where will they reassemble me? Surely such a team is not solely for demolition purposes. They have been too careful, too ordered, too mindful—a well-coordinated plan, efficiently and tenderly carried out.

Yes, I would say that they have been tender with me. I still continue a slow, tedious hobble through my shop when I can, greeting a few friends and even the odd stranger or two. All are aware now. It is uncomfortable to mark their grief. It seems so fresh for them. Why is that? Oh yes, they do not know of the team; they see only the results of their labors. How changed I must be to them—the constant, sturdy shop that has been here since their childhood. Some seem astounded that this would happen, that I would abandon them and be relocated. And yet, can they not see that I am unable even to stand at the counter to talk anymore? I cannot catch up on my rest. It is increasingly hard for me to smile and continue at this game. I will try a little longer, for my family and for my friends, but I must give it up soon. I cannot keep my eyes open for them. I just want to sleep. The gruesome term comes to me: the *sleep of the dead.*

Gruesome? No. I must admit, in fact, that I have found sleep to be refreshingly pleasant as of late. I will not share this knowledge with my family, because their ambitions are now different than mine. I cannot seem to connect with the old shop anymore, and I have been given a gracious peace and, may I say, excitement even, about the "closed for business" sign that will soon be placed on the front door. All interesting items have been removed, and there is little curiosity about the dusty shelves and blank walls. And the sleep—oh the blessed sleep! At first, it was just a disconnection and a wandering, but now, it is so full! Memories connected with dreams! Wonderful, invigorating pictures. The connection pieces are apparently being reassembled, and I am able to drift between the brightness of my dreams, back to the dark shop, and back again to the dream. One foot in two worlds, a life in each day.

There is a persistent shake at my shoulder. My children work to pull me back into the shop. I am reticent, leaving my dream. This one is a beautiful repeat—a bright sun, a canoe resting on a bank, a familiar river. The sun warms pale skin, round pebbles shift under bare feet, a breeze crosses the river in a fleeting zigzag pattern. I am returned completely to my youth. My body is nearly whole again. The canoe and river are hot and cold, sturdy and ...

"Are you awake? Are you okay?" The shaking is insistent, and I find myself lifting up from the riverbank, my body growing heavy and my mind dulling—climbing and grappling, up and away from reality, back into the shop. The fog clamps down in heavy thickness, and I am requested to stand behind the counter again. "Where's the canoe?" I murmur into the dark room, my shop tongue dry and thick.

"He's confused," I hear them say, standing near me at the counter. Yet I am not the confused one. It is very clear what is happening here. But these things cannot be described to others, as I am the owner, and I know the secrets. I desperately want, need, must return to my sleep, my dream. It is required of me. It is my journey, and I wish to take it now. I am anxious and ready. I am a caged animal, ready for its release. The breeze is still in my nostrils, and my desire is for the refreshed energy, the happiness, the wholeness. I don't want to stay and die; I want to go and live.

This trip back to the shop is probably my last. I do not have the strength to turn my head again, to make the climb back out. "Back" is too heavy, too wearying, and ... may we be honest? The shop is empty. Only the last light remains to be turned off, and we will be done here. I open my eyes briefly to see my loved ones peering beseechingly across the counter, but they appear now to be on a different sphere, in an old world ... and I am being made a part of a new world, a more *real* world.

I remain as long as I can for them, making a few, last verbal exchanges, but I think that they cannot hear me from their sphere. I feel a passing of regret that I will not be allowed the final closing of the shop myself, that I will have to leave the turning off of the last light and the hanging of the door sign to others. But it is too difficult to stay here now, clinging to this dream for their sakes. I see tears in many eyes, and I do experience a hurt for them but no feeling of sadness for myself. Their bereaved expressions convey that they feel like they are losing me, but I do not feel that I am losing them. Their world is a dream, and like all dreams, the real feeling just isn't there to feel.

I ponder this for a moment but find my mind blissfully slipping back to my reality—the sun, the breeze, the river, the canoe—in which I am now sitting. And I see that I have floated off the bank a ways. The cloudy feeling of my brain has been released—the fatigue of body and emotions that had clung, fettering me to the old dream, the old world. I am whole and full again and more alive than I have ever been. If only my loved ones could join me here! I wait for the anticipated feeling of sadness at the separation, but it never comes. Just the breeze from the river and the sun in my eyes.

My hand glides down to feel the water. Cool, comforting, delicious. I lay my head back and prop my feet on the crosspiece in front of me, feeling the inner strengthening and consoling that the river has always given me. My youth re-enters me, and there are no words except "All is well."

The canoe meanders placidly to the center of the river, and turning my head, I see the pebbled riverbank recede. There is no need to paddle, nothing to do but absorb and feel. I am being taken to a new life, an older life—different and prior to the one I had lived in my lovely little shop. I experience a comfort of remembered souls and good friends, rest and steadiness, energy and fullness. This ought to feel like death, because I am aware that this is what must have occurred, but it is more like life than anything I have ever felt. Wider and deeper than I have ever known. More complete and more present … a returning and a beginning. A peace that passeth understanding.

QUESTIONS FOR REFLECTION
CHAPTER 6: THE "LOVED ONE"

1. This chapter reverses the viewpoint, reflecting on what dying might feel like from the point of view of "the loved one." The theme repeats itself, that what is seen by the watchers is not necessarily what the one being watched is experiencing. Were you able to place yourself in the shop as a bystander, or did you relate more to the shop owner himself? What disappearing shop items might correlate with the physical changes in our own bodies as we age and eventually "close up shop"?

2. Did you notice that the fatigue and weariness of the shop owner's illness actually helped him come to an acceptance of his terminal condition? What did you feel about the "disassembling" that was described? Have you found that death is simply reckless and undiscriminating or that it has a pattern or a plan of sorts?

3. This story describes a cool river and a warm canoe, a feeling of home and of a place to go. We, of course, don't know exactly what "crossing over" looks like. But we do know that we all die. Do you and your loved one share the same beliefs, and are you able to talk about it openly? If not, how can this be reconciled?

4. This is the last question of the last chapter, and it has been saved for you. Answering for yourself—if you are the shop owner, the "loved one," the one whose head is on the pillow and whose body is on the deathbed ... do you know where you will go when it is your turn to take the journey of one?

(See the gospel story under References.)

REFERENCES

Family Calendar

MONTH:

SUN	MON	TUE	WED	THUR	FRI	SAT
Name Shift	Name Shift	Name Shift	Name Shift	Name Shift	Name Shift	Name Shift
Name Shift	Name Shift	Name Shift	Name Shift	Name Shift	Name Shift	Name Shift
Name Shift	Name Shift	Name Shift	Name Shift	Name Shift	Name Shift	Name Shift

Palliative Performance Scale (PPS)

%	Ambulation	Activity and Evidence of Disease	Self-Care	Intake	Conscious Level
100%	Full	Normal activity No evidence of disease	Full	Normal	Full
90%	Full	Normal activity Some evidence of disease	Full	Normal	Full
80%	Full	Normal activity with effort Some evidence of disease	Full	Normal or reduced	Full
70%	Reduced	Unable to do normal Job / work Some evidence of disease	Full	Normal or reduced	Full
60%	Reduced	Unable to do hobby/ housework Significant disease	Occasional assistance necessary	Normal or reduced	Full or confusion
50%	Mainly sit/lie	Unable to do any work Extensive disease	Considerable assistance required	Normal or reduced	Full or confusion
40%	Mainly in bed	As above	Mainly assistance	Normal or reduced	Full or drowsy or confusion
30%	Totally bedbound	As above	Total care	Reduced	Full or drowsy or confusion
20%	As above	As above	Total care	Minimal sips	Full or drowsy or confusion
10%	As above	As above	Total care	Mouth care only	Drowsy or coma
0	Death				

Note: References are for informational purposes only; they are not intended to diagnose or treat. Please seek professional assistance for interpretation and use.

Karnofsky Performance Status (KPS)

Able to carry on normal activity and to work: no special care needed	100	Normal, no complaints; no evidence of disease
Able to carry on normal activity and to work: no special care needed	90	Able to carry on normal activity; minor signs or symptoms of disease
Able to carry on normal activity and to work: no special care needed	80	Normal activity with effort; some signs or symptoms of disease
Unable to work; able to live at home and care for most personal needs; varying amount of assistance needed	70	Cares for self; unable to carry on normal activity or to do active work
Unable to work; able to live at home and care for most personal needs; varying amount of assistance needed	60	Requires occasional assistance but is able to care for most of his personal needs
Unable to work; able to live at home and care for most personal needs; varying amount of assistance needed	50	Requires considerable assistance and frequent medical care
Unable to care for self; requires equivalent of institutional or hospital care; disease may be progressing rapidly	40	Disabled: requires special care and assistance
Unable to care for self; requires equivalent of institutional or hospital care; disease may be progressing rapidly	30	Severely disabled; hospital admission is indicated although death not imminent
Unable to care for self; requires equivalent of institutional or hospital care; disease may be progressing rapidly	20	Very sick; hospital admission necessary; active support treatment necessary
Unable to care for self; requires equivalent of institutional or hospital care; disease may be progressing rapidly	10	Moribund; fatal processes progressing rapidly
Unable to care for self; requires equivalent of institutional or hospital care; disease may be progressing rapidly	0	Dead

Note: References are for informational purposes only; they are not intended to diagnose or treat. Please seek professional assistance for interpretation and use.

FAST Scale: Functional Assessment Staging Tool for Dementia

Stage	Stage Name	Characteristics	Expected Untreated AD Duration (months)	Mental Age (years)	MMSE (score)
1	Normal aging	No deficits whatsoever	---	Adult	29–30
2	Possible mild cognitive impairment	Subjective functional deficit	---		28–29
3	Mild cognitive impairment	Objective functional deficit interferes with a person's most complex task	84	12+	24–28
4	Mild dementia	IADLs become affected, such as bill paying, cooking, cleaning, traveling	24	8–12	19–20
5	Moderate dementia	Needs help selecting proper attire	18	5–7	15
6a	Moderately severe dementia	Needs help putting on clothes	4.8	5	9
6b	Moderately severe dementia	Needs help bathing	4.8	4	8
6c	Moderately severe dementia	Needs help toileting	4.8	4	5
6d	Moderately severe dementia	Urinary incontinence	3.6	3–4	3
6e	Moderately severe dementia	Fecal incontinence	9.6	2–3	1
7a	Severe dementia	Speaks five to six words during day	12	1.25	0
7b	Severe dementia	Speaks only one word clearly	18	1	0
7c	Severe dementia	Can no longer walk	12	1	0
7d	Severe dementia	Can no longer sit up	12	0.5–0.8	0
7e	Severe dementia	Can no longer smile	18	0.2–0.4	0
7f	Severe dementia	Can no longer hold up head	12+	0–0.2	0

Note: References are for informational purposes only; they are not intended to diagnose or treat. Please seek professional assistance for interpretation and use.

Sharing the Gospel Story with Your Loved One

There are as many ideas about God as there are stars in the heavens. This being said, getting someone to agree with your viewpoint cannot become the main goal. Simply initiate the conversation, and make it safe to continue talking. Break the conversation into several shorter sessions if needed. Though you love this person dearly, his or her decisions about God are not between you and him or her but are between that person and God. Your responsibility is to simply share the story, and let God work on the heart.

Conversation Starter: (Speaking to your loved one)
The doctors have said that your condition is progressing and that there is no cure. I love you, and I want to hear how you feel about meeting God when it's your time. Would you share this conversation with me?

Concept 1
I believe that God loves us and made us to love Him back. Tell me what you think?

Concept 2
I know that your heart is good, and I wish God had set things up so that we all get to be in heaven with Him, but it doesn't look like that's true. If it were, then Jesus wouldn't have had to come to earth at all. Jesus is the bridge that God built for us. He is the invitation. There's no other way to get into God's heaven without *His* bridge. Does this make some sense to you?

Concept 3
Jesus is the greatest love story in the world. Dying for someone else is the deepest way to show them how much you love them. I would take your place right now if I could, to show you how much I love

you. But Jesus doesn't force His way on us; He waits for us to invite Him. Have you let Him in?

Concept 4
Can you tell me your God story? (Listen for a change of heart; see 2 Corinthians 5:17.) If the person doesn't have a true God story, ask permission to pray with him or her that God will show Himself to them. Follow up from here as the person is able and willing.)

Supporting Scriptures
- Concept 1: John 3:16, John 17:3
- Concept 2: Romans 3:23, 2 Thessalonians 1:8–9
- Concept 3: John 1:12, Ephesians 2:8–9, John 3:1–8, Revelation 3:20
- Concept 4: Romans 10:9, 2 Corinthians 5:17

Note from the Author
Thank you for reading this reference; I understand that these concepts will not fit every individual. May God lead us all in our search for truth and the peace that comes with finding it. Amen.

Life Review with Your Loved One

As life comes to a close, there are a few things the dying usually want to hear. They want to know that their life has had value and meaning, that their life counted for something. They want to know from their children's own lips that they will be all right after they are gone. They may want to be forgiven for past wrongs, or they may want to forgive someone. They often want to say thank you, and they almost always want to communicate that they love you. The following conversation starters can help facilitate a life review with your loved one.

Questions for Your Loved One
- Tell me what you miss most about "the good old days."
- Tell me the most significant event of your childhood.
- Tell me about your best friend growing up.
- Tell me about your happiest time.
- Tell me about something you're glad you did, even if it was wrong.
- What do you think was your family's greatest strength?
- Whom are you looking forward to seeing on the other side?
- What matters most to you today?
- What are you most thankful for today?
- Is there anything special that you need to hear from me or that you need me to do?

Your Turn to Share
- I'd like to tell you what I love most about you.
- I'd like to tell you what I learned from you.
- What I will always remember about you is ...
- What I will carry on that came from you is ...
- I'm the most thankful for ...